THE PATIENT FROM HELL

THE
Patient
FROM
Hell

How I Worked with My Doctors to Get the Best of Modern Medicine and How You Can Too

STEPHEN H. SCHNEIDER, PH.D.
With Janica Lane

A MERLOYD LAWRENCE BOOK
LIFELONG BOOKS • DA CAPO PRESS
A Member of the Perseus Books Group

Designed by Brent Wilcox
Set in 11.25 point Berling by The Perseus Books Group

Cataloging-in-Publication data for this book is available from the Library of Congress.

First Da Capo Press edition 2005
ISBN 0-7382-1025-0
ISBN-13 978-0-7382-1025-4

Published by Da Capo Press
A Member of the Perseus Books Group
http://www.dacapopress.com

Da Capo Press books are available at special discounts for bulk purchases in the U.S. by corporations, institutions, and other organizations. For more information, please contact the Special Markets Department at the Perseus Books Group, 11 Cambridge Center, Cambridge, MA 02142, or call (800) 255-1514 or (617) 252-5298, or email special.markets@perseusbooks.com.

1 2 3 4 5 6 7 8 9—09 08 07 06 05

To Dr. Sandra Horning, for saving my life—and for putting up with all my hellish behavior. To the oncology and bone marrow teams at Stanford Hospital for caring and competent practice. To my wife, Terry Root, for taking my illness in stride and for being my advocate, confidant, and best friend. To all my friends and family, for being there for me around the clock when I needed them most.

CONTENTS

Preface: I'm Just a Patient—Doesn't the Doctor Know Best?   ix

CHAPTER 1
"But Doctor, It Takes Three Tests to Find the Bottom"   1

CHAPTER 2
This Better Not Be Serious—I've Got a Plane to Catch   14

CHAPTER 3
Whew! The Tests Are Negative, and I've Got
a Plane to Catch   33

CHAPTER 4
Taking My Lumps: Biopsy Blues   42

CHAPTER 5
"Once per Lethal Disease": Coping with Chemo   67

CHAPTER 6
"How Can You Know I'm in Remission?"   85

CHAPTER 7
What's So Special About Fifty-Five?   109

CHAPTER 8
Graduation to the Bone Marrow Unit   123

CHAPTER 9
Zap It to Me: Staring into a Hiroshima-Dose of Radiation   139

CHAPTER 10
Hospital Arrest   154

CHAPTER 11
My Re-Birthday   171

CHAPTER 12
How Much Risk Is Too Much?   178

CHAPTER 13
Can't I Stay Another Day?   184

CHAPTER 14
Darth Vader in Pink   195

CHAPTER 15
A Delicate Balance   205

CHAPTER 16
Size Matters   213

CHAPTER 17
"In Cancer, Perfect Is Important"   221

CHAPTER 18
"I Think Your Kidneys Did You a Favor"   231

CHAPTER 19
A Successful Partnership   249

CHAPTER 20
You and Your Docs: Allies, Not Adversaries   257

Afterword: A Caregiver's Journey   267
Notes   277
A Guide to Web References   285
Acknowledgments   289
Index   291
About the Authors   300

I'm Just a Patient—
Doesn't the Doctor
Know Best?

This Book Is *Not* Anti-Doctor

On the contrary, the team of medical professionals who treated
me for my cancer at Stanford University Medical Center was ded-
icated, skilled, and caring. I'm still here to tell this story because
they and their research colleagues saved my life. But, as a patient,
I also gained firsthand experience with the system in which these
professionals must maneuver, and I learned that the bureaucracy
and hidebound attitudes embedded in that system are far from
optimal—for doctors or for patients.

This Book *Is* Concerned About Overreliance on "Medicine By the Numbers"

Too often, a patient's treatments are performed "by the book"
rather than being tailored to the patient's specific needs. To put it
more bluntly, much of the care that today's patients receive is
"medicine by the numbers," which is best suited for that mythical
abstraction, the "statistically average patient." Doctors are encour-
aged to rely to a considerable extent on large data sets compiled

from previously completed research and may be discouraged from implementing new techniques until adequate clinical trials have been conducted and data on those trials have been amassed, which can often take a decade or longer.

I do not oppose clinical trials—in fact, I wish clinical trials–based data had been available when I was being treated for my uncommon cancer. Cancer clinical trials are absolutely essential for moving the field forward in the treatment of common cancers, and even more so for uncommon cancers. With childhood cancer, the clinical trials participation rate is near 90 percent, and cure rates are high. With adult cancer, the participation rate is less than 5 percent. This needs to change in order for the triumphs in pediatric cancer treatments to be better achieved at the adult level.

While the data currently available from clinical trials are extremely important for gathering accurate statistics on what works best for the *average* patient, it may be difficult for doctors to extrapolate what the data might mean for nonaverage patients. (And that assumes clinical trials data are actually available; for many cancers, like mine, they hardly yet exist or are only preliminary.) Are you one of these "average" patients? Is *anybody*? Some patients may be fairly similar to this mathematical archetype, in which case "by the book" treatments are probably a good choice, at least as a starting point. Sometimes, particularly for diseases with long histories of successful treatments, going along with the conventional wisdom and standard protocols built from years of data on hundreds or thousands of patients is a reasonable plan. But what if your personal health traits and disease characteristics are nowhere near the mean of the statistical distribution of the many patients before you who participated in clinical trials and allowed their health and treatment information to be entered into the statistical databases?

After being diagnosed with abdominal mesothelioma, a rare and often deadly cancer usually caused by asbestos exposure, the famous paleontologist Stephen Jay Gould discussed being an "outlier" in an enlightening essay entitled "The Median Isn't the Message." In it, he suggested that *most* cancer patients are "outliers": "All evolutionary biologists know that variation itself is nature's only irreducible essence. Variation is the hard reality, not a set of imperfect measures for a central tendency. Means and medians are the abstractions."

If you find that you, too, are an "outlier," then "by the book" treatment is probably not the best option for you, even if it is preferred by your HMO or insurance company. However, most medical institutions are reluctant to pay for costlier new or "unproven" treatments or additional tests that don't fall within the boundaries of commonly used protocols, even if there are good medical reasons to expect that these innovative measures will improve their patients' chances. Frequently this reluctance to innovate is said to be driven by cost-benefit analysis (i.e., the concern that new or unproven treatments may prove costlier than standard protocols), but, as I will show later, such rigid practices can be detrimental economically as well as medically. In fact, considering the results of individualized testing and other data in addition to clinical trials data may provide both health and economic benefits.

How can you know if you are not that mythical average patient, but rather an "outlier"? Individualized testing may help to illuminate any deviations from the norm in your health profile. If such tests do reveal any deviations, then you may very well need individualized care, even if that means your treatment can't be carried out in the conventional or "lowest-cost" manner by your hospital and insurance company. Dealing with these agencies constitutes another potential major battle: If the financial officers in for-profit medical establishments were given a choice between optimal treatments for you and least costs to them, does anyone out there think they would always keep your best interests in mind?

Ironically, it may be up to the patients who have experienced this "medicine by the numbers" up close and personal and have observed that doctors typically rely heavily on—or are compelled to rely on—a fixed set of procedures, many of which are dictated by an institution's private cost-benefit calculations, to spark reforms. A patient's life may depend on such reforms—mine did.

Soap Opera Story or Plea for Change?

My goal here is not just to tell an uplifting, Hollywood-style melodrama of a cancer survivor struggling with his treatments (though it will seem soap opera–esque in some chapters); there are many excellent books that already do that (e.g., *Patient Number One*, Rick Murdock's account of being a medical products CEO with lymphatic cancer;[1] and *It's Not About the Bike*, Lance Armstrong's heroic account of his battle with testicular cancer[2]). My purpose is to uplift in a different sense: to use my cancer treatment experiences to argue for needed reforms in a medical system that I believe is not optimally serving patients—especially those with serious, less-well-studied diseases.

My tale chronicles an isolated case of one persistent, life-threatened patient (that would be me) and his scientist wife; their at-first-skeptical, but soon-to-be-cooperative lead physician; and the collaboration between them that enhanced the likelihood of successful treatment and led to modifications in treatment protocols (procedures) that benefited him and could benefit many other patients. I admit that this sounds like the script for a typical hospital drama:

> Busy but contented professional middle-aged man receives life-shattering diagnosis and then must confront daunting and rigid medical system, endure painful and dangerous treatments, and grapple with many barriers within the hierarchical medical community. Man faces bleak outlook and then—Eureka!—his dogged persistence and an enlightened doctor willing to go beyond conventional methods lead to a happy ending after all, and their cooperative efforts improve treatment for other patients as well.

If there are any high-roller TV or movie agents out there who want the rights to this real-life melodrama, I'm game! However, studio execs would probably insist on cutting out my accounts of the problems with conventional medical statistics, the lack of subjective probabilistic reasoning used by most doctors, and the relative scarcity of individualized testing and protocols that I believe could substantially improve outcomes—and these are the most important messages of my story. I am confident that these messages will prove to be important at both the individual (patient) and the institutional (medical establishment) level.

This story will report how a nondoctor can help design his or her own treatment, and I hope that other sufferers of serious illnesses and their friends, families, and professional advocates will use this book as a tool for working with their doctors to do just that. All quotes are our best recollection of such conversations. I'll explain how to negotiate better with doctors and become a full partner in your treatment design, how to seek better treatments that may not fall within standard practice, how to survive difficult hospital procedures, and how to obtain access to nonstandard, individualized pre- or posttreatment diagnostics—one of the most critical and too-often lacking elements of cancer treatments around the world.

A Sobering Global Perspective

It is unquestionable that we're much healthier today because of medicine and its continuous advances, but there are still countless unmet health needs around the world. In the United States, the world's largest economy, 40 to 50 million people in a population of nearly 300 million lack medical insurance; in the world in general, more than 50 percent of people have little or no access to health care. So why focus on individualizing treatments for "dread diseases" in developed nations, a health care issue involving only an elite segment of the world's population?

While I agree that we certainly cannot forget about the AIDS epidemics in Africa and Asia, the age-old battles with tuberculosis and malaria in many developing nations, and other global health problems, the importance of addressing those issues is no reason to rule out striving for reform in first-world hospitals. Effecting a revolution in treatment procedures in these establishments may be more easily attainable, especially given that a treatment regime tailored to an individual patient may be more effective and only marginally more costly (and sometimes cheaper) than following a standard practice. If modern medical institutions can bring themselves to realize that a patient's chances of survival could increase dramatically if spending on that patient's treatments rose from, say, $300,000 to $305,000 (less than 2 percent), a revolution in first-world health care could ensue.

Focusing on medicine in the United States and in other economically strong countries with high levels of technology does not mean ignoring the need to deliver health care to the less-privileged billions in the forgotten world. Once this idea of individualization becomes a brighter blip on the health care establishment's screen, it is my hope that the benefits of patient-based treatments will spill over to help the neediest patients as well.

The Doctor Knows Best?

Confronting the rules, regulations, and hierarchical structures inherent in most hospitals is intimidating enough for any ordinary person, let alone one numbed by a terrible diagnosis. Thus, most physicians—and patients—act as if the patient's role is simply to take orders and be cooperative. Tradition suggests that only medical experts should decide on what treatment course to take; patients are presumed both incapable of material contribution to such decisions and likely to have a poorer prognosis if they are even made aware of the dark side of treatment.

But sometimes the patient knows better, at least about how the patient feels and what the patient needs. By facing the hospital bureaucracy and convincing doctors to individualize diagnostic tests and reexamine some conventional treatment practices, a patient may be able to improve his or her chances of survival. Based on my own four-year, still-successful fight with an uncommon blood cancer, mantle cell lymphoma, I am convinced that my persistence and my insistence on partnering with my doctors in redesigning several aspects of my medical treatment, rather than just picking from a short menu of standard protocols, has contributed to my continuing survival. The feistiness you may observe in me as my story unfolds not only helped me form a partnership with my doctors, it also allowed me to emerge from my cancer experiences with high energy and a fighting spirit.

To Read or Not to Read?

Understanding ahead of time what one is likely to go through while being treated for a dread disease can help eliminate the fear of the unknown. Knowing that I got through it and am still doing OK might help some of you who have recently received a serious diagnosis to overcome the fear and depression that commonly accompany it. The tales of heroic struggle in the Armstrong and Murdock books did this for me.

But be forewarned that my approach is not for everyone. If you're a person who'd rather have full faith in your medical team, who would not deal well with knowing all the "warts" of treatment, who would become particularly disturbed on discovering the array of errors that are too often committed in hospitals, or who would get too angry learning that treatments are often dictated by immediate costs rather than long-term cost-effectiveness, social costs, and the patient's well-being, then simply don't read on. If the kind of information, some of it not terribly reassuring, that I'm going to present is going to dishearten you, please put down the book. Keeping your stress levels down during treatment is hard enough, and knowing "too much" about the reality of your situation may or may not make it worse; you can decide that for yourself. But, a loved one, friend, or professional medical advocate could always absorb what I'll report and tell it to you as needed or serve as your liaison.

If, on the other hand, you think you can stomach some pretty unpleasant details about cancer treatments and the way medicine is sometimes practiced, read on. Continue on to my story if you want to know the pros and cons of treatment alternatives and want to play a major role in treatment decisions. This book will help you choose *for yourself* how to weigh different kinds of risks and make smart trade-offs rather than have others choose for you, often without your even knowing what's at stake. If you want to learn how to take intelligent risks, how to determine whether the cure is worse than the disease or vice versa, this detailed account of my four years of experiences with non-Hodgkin's lymphoma may help you. If you want to surmount the bureaucratic obstacles and financial impediments that often stand in the way of obtaining the best treatments, please read carefully—and if you agree with me, you, too, can take action to help change the status quo. I particularly hope that physicians and public health specialists who agree with me can use my book to help push for needed changes in their institutions—which they know how to do much better than I.

The benefits of becoming involved in your treatment may extend well beyond your particular case. In fact, some of the modifications to typical protocols I negotiated for myself are now being administered to other patients at Stanford University Medical Center, providing evidence that being a full partner in your treatment can help not only you but perhaps your medical professionals and fellow patients as well. This model of patient-as-team-member needs to spread far beyond Stanford University Medical Center, a teaching hospital with a world-class reputation, especially for its lymphoma research.

Even at a research hospital like Stanford, it was at first hard to be taken seriously as a patient partner. You, too, will find that it takes tenacity and effort to learn enough about your illness, the pros and cons of conventional treatment, and where the cutting edge of research lies, especially if you have a rare disease. There are groups out there that can help, such as specialized support groups, the Leukemia and Lymphoma Society of America, and other disease advocacy groups, but ultimately it is your fight (see the Guide to Web References, page 285).

Although blind faith may be comfortable for you as a patient, if you are willing to stick your neck out, you or someone you feel comfortable having act as your advocate can assess the sometimes treacherous trade-offs available to you and chart your own course—and you may very well maximize your chances for cure or remission at the same time.

Who Am I?

First, you need to know a little bit more about me, who I am and who I am not. I'm not a physician, nor do I have an iota of medical training. But, I *am* a doctor—more precisely, I have a doctorate in plasma physics—and I have been studying the Earth's climate for more than thirty years. I'm a professor of biological sciences and a senior fellow at the Institute for International Studies at Stanford University—and, by the way, I have had no formal training in biology *or* international studies. As a climatologist working on the controversial and uncertainty-riddled field of global warming (in which I had no formal training either), I'm well aware of where scientific expertise ends and personal value judgments begin. The expertise that we scientists have to offer— to politicians, citizens, the media, and other scientists—lies in assessments about the range of outcomes that can happen in a given situation and the probabilities that each of those possible outcomes will occur. But determining how to act in the face of such risks (e.g., enacting policies on adaptation to or mitigation of climate change, promoting efficient hybrid vehicles, subsidizing users of alternative energy, or ignoring the problem altogether) involves not science but political or personal value judgments.

Two knowledgeable scientists in the same field, for example, could reach the same scientific conclusion but have very different personal views about how to respond to it. In global warming, I can claim schooled knowledge about the likelihood of rising sea levels, of intensified storms, heat waves, and wildfires, and of climate-related alteration of natural and human systems. However, deciding on whether to invest current resources (and how much or who pays) to reduce possible future risks is not science but a value judgment about how to make trade-offs and how to share the burden of mitigating such risks. I have long believed that "coin-flip" (50–50) odds of significant, planetary scale, and perhaps catastrophic, changes resulting from our using the atmosphere as an unpriced dump for our gaseous waste products, like carbon dioxide, is too high to ignore and should be dealt with by considering mitigation and adaptation policies. Indeed, we buy insurance against improbable disasters when the odds are much lower than this. But this is my personal value judgment, not science, and others may or may not be in agreement with it.

Medical Roulette

Surprisingly, a global problem like climate change, I learned, turns out to be very similar to many personal medical situations. As I became increasingly involved in the decisions related to my own cancer treatments, I realized that my life's work in climate science and policy provided me with remarkably useful background for performing such assessments. Like climate science, medicine entails ascertaining what might happen with or without intervention—in this case treatment; what various treatments might do to alleviate certain conditions; what side effects might be generated by the treatments; and how the roulette wheel is set up—that is, what probability of success can be assigned to each alternative. And here's where the role of patient-as-partner comes in: It's up to you to decide with your doctors what treatment options are best for you and whether or not the side effects of the "cure" are worth it given the probability of success; it's not just an expert judgment. Let me repeat: *Choosing what risks to take is not a medical decision.* You will be qualified to make choices about how you wish to face these risks once you know the range of potential outcomes and estimates of their likelihoods.

You'll actually be doing your doctors a favor if you relieve them of the burden of selecting treatments for you. Discuss the probabilities and consequences of the various options regarding your illness and treatments with them as well as with your friends, family, or advocate, and then decide how you want to face the medical roulette wheel. After all, it is you who, for better or worse, will be cured, become sicker, and suffer side effects. If you learn enough about the range of options, standard or not, available to you, and if you can set up a cooperative partnership with your doctors to best exploit those options, thereby individualizing your treatment, you might rig the medical roulette wheel more in your favor. You can learn from books, from the World Wide Web, and, of course, from your doctors. I hope you can also learn from this book.

It's About You, Not Them

Once again, most doctors are neither ignorant, nor malevolent, nor money-grubbing, nor uncaring. Virtually everyone in the medical profession with whom I have dealt, both during my cancer treatments and well before that, has genuinely wanted the best outcomes for me and my loved ones and all their patients, which also tend to be the best outcomes for their reputations. I am still very thankful to my doctors for being open to my endless questioning, which eventually led to the modification of otherwise fixed practices, the individualization of diagnostic testing and treatments, and the improvement of my chances of survival, although it is still not guaranteed. While this battle with my disease may never be over, I believe my odds are vastly better than they would have been if my doctors had rigidly insisted on treatments "by the book."

With a little prodding from you or your advocate, your doctors and their support staffs will likely teach you a great deal about your situation. However, just remember that many of them are stuck in a cost-conscious and tradition-bound medical system that discourages accommodation of individual patient needs by deviating from standard methods of diagnosis and treatment. It is a very hierarchical profession; status counts, and the patient is usually near the bottom rung of the status ladder.

If you are not willing to accept being treated as the "average patient" or you are facing a less-well-studied disease for which clinical trials or other data to guide a medical regimen are scarce, then fighting your disease will likely require thinking outside the box. It is important that your physicians use all available knowledge on processes, outcomes, and probabilities to select the treatments that appear to provide the greatest chances of success for you—even if an uncomfortably large amount of uncertainty remains. Such "deep uncertainty" is not ideal but must be confronted regardless. Creative thinking and individualized testing can often substitute for limited data, and they are essential when extensive historical data aren't available.

In many aspects of our lives, we act in the face of uncertainty. Techniques for assessing problems that lack massive historical databases of information not only exist but are practiced all over the world by businesses, defense departments, environmental research teams, and other organizations facing complex problems that must be acted on before all of the uncertainties surrounding them can be resolved. However, this decision-analysis approach is all too rare in medical practice, in my view. Let's change that. Get informed about your disease, get involved in your treatment, and insist on choosing how to deal with your own risks. Good luck—your life could depend on it!

1 "But Doctor, It Takes Three Tests to Find the Bottom"

I WAS SCARED TO DEATH. Dr. Sandra Horning, a renowned oncologist at Stanford University Medical Center and the main doctor treating my cancer, was writing up the final orders for my chemotherapy, which was scheduled to begin a few hours later. I felt perfectly healthy despite the clear medical diagnostics to the contrary, which I had seen and heard myself. It was all very surreal; could it really be me with those grim pathology reports and lumpy CT and PET scans? The only thing that felt different was that I had a few swollen lymph nodes, and they didn't really hurt, but I knew I couldn't continue to deceive myself. I was well aware from my research on the Web that without the chemo treatments, I probably wouldn't live out the year. But still, it seemed strange to think that in a few more chimes of the clock, I, a perfectly healthy-feeling person, was going to be poisoned. And I had agreed to it!

It Takes Three

In a fearful situation, nothing centers me more than an unanswered question to explore. I switch into analytical mode and get comfortable again. Indeed, that's what happened as I was finishing my examination and consultation in the oncology wing at Stanford Hospital and preparing for chemotherapy. The oncology Fellow (a Fellow is a doctor undergoing further specialized training after completing residency training) handed me chemo orders for that afternoon, along with a separate yellow sheet that I was to bring back in another eleven days, on August 20, 2001, when I was scheduled for a blood test. Not loving the idea of yet more invasive needle pokes, I asked, "Why the test?" hoping secretly that it would be for some frivolous reason and I could talk them out of it. "It's to find your nadir," the Fellow explained quickly, heading toward the door to the waiting room, where a throng of other anxious cancer patients sat. "What's my nadir?" I asked. "Your low point. The chemicals used in the chemotherapy kill not only your fast-growing lymphoma cells but also the good cells you need in order for your immune system to fully function." "So the nadir is my white blood cell count's lowest value after the chemo?" I questioned, feeling oh-so-much less frightened as my left brain reverted to its normal dominant position. "Exactly," he said, moving closer to the door. "But how do you know I'll reach my nadir exactly eleven days from now?" I persisted. "Well, most patients' white blood cell counts bottom out in about eleven days. Your body will detoxify the chemo chemicals in a few days, and then your white blood cell count will drop for about a week, bottom out in the second week, and begin recovering in the third week. Then we'll hit you with the next round of chemo." He moved back into the room, seeming to enjoy teaching me and my wife, Terry Root, the basics.

"How important is it for you to know my nadir?" I asked. "Extremely important. If it's very low—a white count below 500 per microliter [normal is 3,800–10,000, and *my* normal was about 4,800]—your immunity could be so compromised that even a common bacterial infection like bronchitis could be devastating, or bacteria that your body can normally hold in check, like that in your digestive tract, could grow out of control."

"Can you draw for me in the air what a typical white count cycle looks like between chemos?" The Fellow traced out a bowl-like curve, with a straight-line decrease representing the first week, followed by a U-shaped dip for the second week, and then an upward recovery of the white blood cells in the third week—not back to normal, but certainly not dangerously immune-compromised. "So the nadir occurs in the second week in the parabola you drew?" "Right, that's typical." "But how can you draw a parabola with only one data point? Won't I need three blood tests to assure we don't miss the nadir?" By this time, I was no longer thinking about getting out of another "ghouling"—my term for blood draws—but in fact wanted to add two more to be sure they really found my nadir. The mathematical principle that states that three points are needed to draw any parabola apparently was neglected in the diagnostic treatment plan.

"Doing the blood test eleven days after chemo is just what we do—you know, a rule of thumb. Actually, some docs don't do the nadir test at all and just treat patients with antibiotics if they get sick," the Fellow explained as he turned back to the door, presuming I understood the protocol. I didn't let up: "But you could easily miss the bottom." "It's just how it's done. Don't worry; it will give us the information we need." His chemo lesson was over, and there were indeed many patients waiting who also needed the skills of these medics if they were to have a chance at life, so I gave up—for a few minutes, anyway.

As I was signing out of the Oncology Day Care Center and the reality of having an IV feeding toxic chemicals into my body was twenty minutes closer, I noticed that the nurse who had scheduled my blood test was gone, and there was a different nurse in the area. I had a flash: "Excuse me," I said to the nurse, "I was told to get a blood test on August 17. Could you schedule it for me?" "Of course." She went to the computer, and after I gave her my code numbers, she entered the appointment into my record. That meant I had a computer order for a blood test on August 17 to go along with my paper order for a test on August 20. As I checked out, I asked the nurse, "Who else could authorize a blood test?" "The doctor's nurse practitioner," I was told. I picked up the practitioner's card, and she got a phone call from me a few days later: "Sorry to bother you," I said, "but I was told to get a blood test on August 23, after my chemo. Could you put the order into the computer for me?" "Sure." I heard the clicking of her fingers on her keyboard, and a few seconds later, she said, "Done." "Many thanks," I said, rather pleased with myself for having so easily gamed the system and found a way to get my three data points.

After spending days thinking about how horrible my first chemo session was going to be, I found that the aftereffects weren't nearly as bad as I'd expected—although it was no fun *while* it was happening, as I'll explain in chapter 5. However, the first chemo session is always rumored to be the least difficult because the patient's immune system is still largely intact then. I could only imagine how the next few rounds would be. But let's get back to my three data points, since it will make a much larger point about "medicine by the numbers."

When August 17 rolled around, I popped into Oncology Day Care to get ghouled. Several hours later, I got a phone call from a nurse telling me that my white blood cell count was below normal—around 2,100 per microliter—but that at this level my risk of infection was not very high. I was told merely to be careful to avoid people who were obviously sick.

Three days later, shortly after I had gone to Oncology Day Care with the yellow sheet for my regularly scheduled blood test (my *second* blood test), I got a phone call from another nurse telling me that my white count was somewhere around 600 per microliter and that I needed to be quite careful to avoid sick people, but that this level wasn't so dangerous that I would be at high risk of a serious infection—pneumonia is a common one, as are intestinal problems—from my own body's natural bacteria. There was also a risk of neutropenia, which is when the level of neutrophils—the mature white blood cells that account for 50 to 70 percent of all white blood cells and are disease- and infection-fighters—becomes very low, increasing the risk of microbial illness. My neutrophil count was pretty low—below 500 (normal is anywhere from 1,500 to 8,000)—but at least my overall white blood cell count was above 500.

I asked whether it was safe to attend a wedding for one of Terry's graduate students. The nurse said, "Sure, particularly if it's outside, you don't share food, and you wash your hands with alcohol disinfectant frequently." I dutifully followed her instructions, enjoyed the wedding, and didn't suffer any health-related disasters.

Fourteen days after my chemo, on August 23, after having gone in for my *third* blood test, I was back at work in my office on the Stanford campus when my private line rang. "Schneider," I answered. "Dr. Schneider, I'm calling from the Stanford Oncology Day Care Center. Are you in your office?" the voice on the other end of the line asked, her intonation suggesting that I shouldn't be. "Yes, I was told that was all right." "Well, your blood test shows that you have a very low neutrophil count and a white count near 500. You're in grave danger of serious infection. In fact, you might be better off being in the hospital and on prophylactic [preventive] antibiotics." "Hospital? Isn't that the place where the germs congregate? Can you check with Dr. Horning to make sure that that's what she thinks I ought to do? I promise I'll stay in my office and avoid contact with anyone." About half an hour later, she called back and said, "Dr. Horning says that you don't need to come to the hospital. Just go home and stay there. Avoid people and animals for the next five days."

I reluctantly told Françoise Fleuriau-Halcomb, my administrative assistant at the time, to cancel all my appointments, have people call me at home, and cross her fingers that using the lousy telephone modem on my laptop to establish a connection to the Internet wouldn't frustrate me to death as I tried to keep up with e-mail at home. I tried to act calm, but I guess I *was* pretty nervous about coming in contact with harmful germs in the office or at home, or, even more frightening, developing a serious disease from my own, naturally occurring bacteria. But Sandra suggested that I didn't even need prophylactic antibiotics if I stayed away from people, so I took a deep breath and tried to keep my cool as I biked home, unaware that riding through the dust clouds generated by the construction projects on campus was potentially dangerous. As I was later told, the fungi in that dust could have been enough to cause a life-threatening fungal lung infection in a person with a white blood cell count of 500. Fortunately, nothing happened.

Housebound?

The five days at home, my first bout of "house arrest," occurred before classes had started at Stanford for the 2001–2002 school year, so I could be almost as productive at home as in my office on campus, although I generally believe that face-to-face meetings with colleagues and students are more effective than phone calls. However, the prospect of having to miss a week of work every three weeks (when I reached my nadir after chemo) once I had started teaching classes for the autumn quarter was not one I relished, nor would my students and colleagues, although they would surely understand. I was still working full time despite suffering some side effects from chemo, and I had no intention of backing out of my professional life, aside from staying off airplanes, which could be death traps for me, given all the germs that float around in the confined spaces of their cabins. In fact, I had rationalized to myself, staying off airplanes might actually allow me to catch up on some of my backlog of work, write some papers, and interact more with my students. But to be made to stay home for one week of every three, especially when I felt almost fine, was going to be very difficult.

Terry, too, was distraught about my low white blood cell count and consequent solitary confinement. She had spent countless hours researching lymphoma on the Web, and she found out that a new drug called Neupogen, produced by the biotechnology company Amgen, was supposed to be very effective at stimulating stem cells to produce white blood cells after chemotherapy, thereby enhancing immunity. We wondered why I hadn't been given a prescription for Neupogen immediately after my first chemo session. The accounts we read on the Web suggested that it was quite effective in keeping chemo patients with my kind of treatment—specifically designed to kill B cells (since my cancer was a B-cell type)—at safer white blood cell count levels by stimulating their stem cells to produce noncancerous B cells. (Stem cells presumably produce only benign cells; cancer cells reproduce themselves once they are present. Of course, there is controversy about this too, which we'll discuss later.) Treatment with Neupogen might allow me to stay permanently above the 500 white count level, even after very harsh rounds of chemotherapy.

—┤├—

Finally, my nadir week ended, and my white count was presumed to be recovering, so I went back to work, although I was still careful to avoid anyone who looked sniffly. Precisely three weeks after my first chemotherapy, I returned to the Stanford Oncology Day Care Center to be examined and to begin my second chemo treatment. The doctors, looking through my records, presumably caught on to my gaming stunt of getting the three blood tests, but nobody mentioned it. We just discussed my very low white blood cell count, and I resisted a churlish "I told you so."

Does the Test Tell You What You Need to Know?

The single blood test is just one of many examples in medicine of a standard procedure that is outdated, inaccurate, or inconclusive and/or is based mainly on cost considerations, which can limit the amount of potentially useful information available and ultimately result in poorer care for the patient involved. There are countless examples in oncology and nearly all other fields of medicine of tests not being given, even if the results of such tests might give doctors and patients more and better information. In addition, many tests are avoided until "absolutely necessary," at which point it is possible that less effective—and in the long run, perhaps more expensive—means of detection and treatment will have to be pursued. Later, I'll again relate this back to my cancer.

On a more optimistic note, there are many instances in which the "right" tests are performed as standard procedure. In preventive medicine, for example, there are detailed guidelines on the age at which people should have screening tests such as those for blood pressure, cholesterol levels, cervical cancer, breast cancer, prostate cancer, colorectal cancer, hearing, and eyesight—as well as how often. Such tests tend to be fairly reliable, and although some are expensive up front, they may prevent serious health problems and much greater treatment costs later.

Many diagnostic tests also tell doctors and patients what they need to know. When a patient comes in with a suspicious-looking mole or other irregular skin coloration, if cancer is a possibility, a skin biopsy is the first step taken. The results are conclusive; the test typically gives a yes or no answer. Similarly, when a patient is thought to have a serious blood disorder, a bone marrow biopsy (which I will describe in chapter 5) is often among the first tests performed, and the results can usually be used to make a diagnosis, or at least to rule out many nasty possibilities.

The difficulty for patients or their advocates is in distinguishing between tests that tell them what they need to know and tests that don't tell them enough. Medicine is constantly improving, and we can expect that there will be fewer and fewer examples of inaccurate or insufficient tests out there as a result, but in the meantime we have to be diligent in considering what is being done and what a test will or won't tell us. Don't be afraid to ask your doctors why they are ordering certain tests and not ordering others.

—┤ ├—

Back at the hospital, I was given another yellow sheet for a blood test, and this time it was to take place fourteen days after my next chemo treatment rather than eleven. I wasn't told to come in for three separate blood tests, but at least my test date had been moved back so that it corresponded with where my nadir would likely be—a perfect example of what is called "Bayesian updating," the constant revising of a theory, procedure, or opinion as new data become available. (I'll explain the value of this approach in more detail in chapter 2.) I decided not to challenge the decision to perform a single blood test a few days later in the chemo cycle, figuring I could once again manipulate the system over the phone if necessary.

To Override or Not to Override?

After my appointment at the Oncology Day Care Center, Terry and I walked up to the chemo ward, where the very competent nurses put an IV into my arm, which by this time was already so routine that I hardly felt it. Then they gave me some very potent antinausea drugs and an IV dose of Benadryl, which, in pill form, is a standard over-the-counter antihistamine. It's amazing that a 25 milligram pill of Benadryl taken orally typically causes only mild drowsiness, but 25 milligrams in a drip bag elicits extreme grogginess, akin to wearing a chain mail suit. The nurses explained to me that the amount of Benadryl the human body absorbs from a pill is far less than the full 25 milligrams, whereas the IV delivery assures that every last drop enters the bloodstream. I asked why I needed the Benadryl. The answer was that some patients are allergic to the chemotherapy they are given, and the Benadryl would minimize any allergic reaction one might have. I figured that being half knocked out probably also helped people tolerate the treatment process, so I didn't mind it at all.

Three weeks earlier, my chemo session had begun ten or fifteen minutes after the nurses administered the Benadryl. This time, more than an hour and a half had gone by, and I was beginning to wonder what was happening. My Benadryl-induced haze didn't stop my brain from saying, *This is different; what's going on?* I heard my name bouncing back and forth in a conversation between some nurses standing about thirty feet away. That immediately lifted my chain mail, and I listened very carefully. "I guess we'll have to send him home," one said. A few minutes later, a nurse came in and explained that my blood test that day had shown a white count of only 1,600 cells per microliter and that the hospital's standard protocol dictated that it be higher for the chemo to be dispensed. "But Dr. Horning told me I have to be religious about doing the chemotherapy every three weeks exactly," I protested. "I don't want to wait another few days for my white cell count to increase, because the cancer count will go up too!" "Well, because your white cell count has not rebounded to safe levels, proceeding with the chemo treatment will likely drive it down to dangerously low levels. These are the rules we have to follow." "I'm not going anywhere," I said. "Please talk to Dr. Horning and find out if she wants me to go through with the chemo or not."

The one thing Sandra Horning had made abundantly clear when she originally designed my chemo regimen was that I should not delay my chemotherapy treatments. "These chemos drive down your cancer, and the fact that you had a very low white count is actually good news," she had said earlier that morning, "since it means that while the chemotherapy drugs were killing the good guys, they were also killing the bad guys." It was consoling to know that I was at least getting something good out of taking this risk. "I don't want you to delay your treatment, because as your good cells begin to grow back after chemo, so does the cancer, and we want to keep hitting it and hitting it again and hitting it again," she explained. It all made good sense.

About half an hour later, an oncology Fellow came upstairs and explained that Dr. Horning did not want me to leave, and in fact she had insisted that they go ahead with the chemo so that no time would be lost in the fight against my dread disease. She obviously had authority to overrule the protocol, and I was highly appreciative of that. In addition, Dr. Horning suggested I be given a prescription for Neupogen so that my white count would remain within the safe zone in the weeks after chemo. (Neupogen stimulates production of neutrophils, white blood cells that attack bacteria and viruses. It does nothing for the B cells themselves.) Terry, remembering her Web reading, asked, "Why didn't Steve get Neupogen in the first place?" "You have to earn it," the Fellow explained. "Earn it?" I asked incredulously. "Yes. If your white count doesn't fall to 500, then we don't administer Neupogen, but since yours dropped to that level, you are now authorized to take it. We prescribe Neupogen only when patients' blood tests prove it necessary; only 20 percent of patients ever end up needing it." My left brain kicked in: "Well, if you did three blood tests on each patient after every chemotherapy session, maybe you'd find that 40 or 50 percent of them would 'earn it' rather than 20 percent," I said. I was not a happy camper, and I don't think the Fellow was either after being boxed in by my suggestion that the hospital's procedures weren't optimal. I was, however, pleased that the hospital was using Bayesian updating to some degree, as evidenced by the decision to administer Neupogen based on my earlier postchemo white blood cell counts.

"How much do these Neupogen shots cost?" I asked. The Fellow wasn't sure, but he thought it was something on the order of $300 each, and I would have to take five of them in the week after chemo. "So, just to save the hospital or my insurance company $1,500, I was put at higher risk of neutropenia and other infections and was forced to stay home from work for a week, which amounted to a loss to myself and to Stanford of well over $1,500?" I asked. "It's just the cost-benefit ratio the hospital uses," he said. That comment caused my left brain to override the Benadryl haze; I was back in fighting form. "In cost-benefit terminology, economists define a cost as the sum of private *plus* social costs [a social cost in this case would be the lost economic value to Stanford from my not being there for a week, for example]. All this hospital is doing is minimizing its immediate private costs and not considering what is socially beneficial and therefore what is most economically efficient. It's just bad economics and shortsighted self-interest. Add what the cost would've been to my insurance, the hospital, and my body if an infection had developed, and the withholding of Neupogen could've been a very expensive mistake."

I wasn't angry at the Fellow, but I was beginning to get frustrated with "the system." I realized that "medicine by the numbers" not only was dangerous for me but also was holding the Fellow back. First, the hospital's standard procedure had called for only one blood test when three were clearly necessary, at least the first time around. The third blood test, which I had surreptitiously scheduled for myself, was the one that revealed the dangerously low white count that "earned" me Neupogen, the white blood cell stimulant. Then "the numbers" said that my white count was too low for me to go through with my second scheduled chemo session—and my best interests were served only by having that "by-the-book" rule overruled by Dr. Horning. And, finally, it was becoming clear that the hospital's bureaucrats did not have their cost-benefit numbers even remotely right, and as a result I was almost denied Neupogen, a drug I very much needed.[1]

The Costs of Medicine By the Book

While it is clear that medical professionals must adhere to well-defined, standardized rules and ethical procedures, mainly to ensure the well-being of their patients, some discrepancies exist between performing medicine by the book and doing what is best for the patient, as my examples above illustrate and as you will see throughout this book. The danger in this approach is threefold: 1) Poor tests and testing methods may fail to show that a patient is in danger, as would have been the case with me had it not been for the three blood tests. 2) Faulty cost-benefit analyses can deny patients drugs they need, which can lead to many risks, including additional health problems, missed time at work, and so on. 3) These flaws in "the system" may cost medical institutions far more than the cost of the drug or the extra tests and, multiplied by thousands of patients, could cause long-term financial hemorrhage.

Back in the infusion chair, Benadryl and all, I began to muse that decision analysis, cost-benefit methods, and other analytic tools that we use all the time in environmental science and policy seemed to be sorely lacking—or at least poorly applied—in medicine. Before the chain mail suit completely descended again, I thought to myself, *I may need to write a book about this*.

—|—

But let me now start at the beginning. The remainder of this book details my experiences with mantle cell lymphoma in chronological order. Some chapters span days, others weeks or months, and the final two, years. This is perhaps a decent analogy for my cancer struggle: There were—and there continue to be—up days and down days, with the up days passing at lightning speed and the down days dragging on for what seem like weeks on end. I have learned tremendously from both the positives and the negatives, and throughout this book I will impart this information to you in the hopes that you will be even better prepared than I was to step into the ring and battle your condition.

2 | This Better Not Be Serious—I've Got a Plane to Catch

W HY DID IT ALWAYS have to be like this before I headed out of town? Addressing everything that had been piling up on my desk, filling my e-mail inbox, and cluttering my head for weeks always got jammed into the last two days before a flight, which meant two five-hour nights of sleep and the consequent disruption of normal circadian rhythms, a groggy head, and the feeling of jet lag before even boarding the jet. I've only done this about 1,500 times, so by now you'd think I'd know how to do it without stress. No such luck.

On that particular morning in February 2001, I was already awake and didn't even need the alarm to jostle me out of sleep; intrusive thoughts kept jamming into my head, shortening my already shortened night. How were we going to sell 300 representatives of 100 governments attending the Intergovernmental Panel on Climate Change (IPCC) plenary meeting in Geneva, Switzerland, on the idea that global warming was not just a theory but already could be shown to be influencing the behaviors and movements of plants and animals all around the world? Terry had been working on this problem for over five years, and I knew she'd have to sit up on the dais at the plenary meeting addressing some skeptical delegates, who, despite being in the diplomatic corps of their countries' governments, were anything but diplomatic when it came to making meaningful decisions and tackling delicate issues affecting their national interests.

Having had a hand in Terry's research, I'd be up there too, and I was mulling over how I could deflect the more obstreperous remarks that I was certain would come from the representatives of oil-producing countries like Saudi Arabia and the other OPEC nations. At meeting after meeting, these representatives were as disruptive as possible, refusing to accept the seriousness of climate science, since it might lead to calls for a "cure" to global warming that involved increasing the efficiency with which we use fossil fuels as well as a major increase in the use of renewable, sustainable energy. A global shift away from burning fossil fuels would cost these countries trillions of dollars, so how could anyone expect them to embrace wholeheartedly the global warming problem?

Then there were the developing countries, who saw the rich countries—the United States, Japan, and the Western European countries, for example—as having gotten wealthy over the past century and a half by using the atmosphere as a giant free dump for their tailpipe and smokestack emissions. As these developing nations began to industrialize, increase output, and improve the material well-being of their citizens, they perceived that the rich nations had invented new obstacles—global warming, the greenhouse effect, and policies to cope with them—only to block their progress, keep them behind economically, and prevent them from enjoying the fruits of the same industrialization the developed nations had used to get rich. Their concerns are understandable but dangerous for the planet. The atmosphere probably couldn't easily absorb worldwide per capita emissions equal to those of the United States or Europe, particularly since the developing world has four times the "capita" (population) of the rich countries. But the developing nations were not going to act without help from the rich countries, which have created 80 percent of the global warming problem so far.

The first step before tackling these huge issues was to wake up and get going. I figured a hot shower would be a good way to make myself feel a little more human. The hot water is welcoming on cold, early mornings, especially those preceded by near-sleepless nights. That morning in the shower, as I raised my right arm and prepared to soap myself with my left hand, I noticed a star-shaped black and blue mark on the inside of my upper right arm, about two inches above my elbow. I wondered how I had ended up with the strange mark; I didn't remember banging myself. *No matter*, I thought. But as I applied the soap and the fingers of my left hand slid smoothly over the slippery, soapy skin of my right arm, I felt something a little funny. It was almost imperceptible at first, so I very lightly ran my fingertips down my arm below my right armpit again, and, sure enough, the area seemed to be slightly swollen. I tried the same thing in the same place on my left arm, and it wasn't swollen. I went back to my right arm, started to feel around some more, and soon found what felt like a BB in the center of the puffiness. A flash of worry came across me, and I thought, *Oh no, I hope this isn't phlebitis.*[1] I've got a plane to catch in six hours and a class to teach in two.

A few years earlier Terry had had a similar black and blue mark and a lump in her armpit, which turned out to be phlebitis. There was a clot blocking a vein in her armpit, and it took two days of hospitalization and anticoagulation drugs to disintegrate the clot and make sure it didn't move somewhere more dangerous, like her lungs. I also remembered having to inject her with anticoagulants once she came home from the hospital, which wasn't fun for either of us.

Although I was concerned that the bump could be serious, all I could think was that I couldn't afford to lose a couple of days at any time, much less as we were about to head off to Geneva. I had worked for three years, for hours every day, on getting the report prepared for the IPCC meeting, and everything depended on the five-day Geneva plenary meeting. I *had* to be there.

I agonized over what to do. Should I call Michael Jacobs, my internist at Stanford University Medical Center, or just sneak out of the country and pretend the bump wasn't there? I almost certainly would have chosen the latter, except that I couldn't lie to Terry, and if I mentioned the bump and the black and blue mark to her while we were in Geneva and she found out I hadn't called Michael, she would very likely have tried to pressure me into heading back home immediately, especially after her own scare with phlebitis. So when I emerged from the shower, fully awake now (and not just from the hot water), I talked with Terry and she confirmed that I should call Michael. I got hold of Michael's nurse practitioner and explained the urgency of talking to Michael directly; twenty-five minutes later, the phone rang.

"Is there any streaking along the inside of your arm?" Michael asked. I figured he was checking for phlebitis or some type of poisoning, neither of which was particularly comforting. "No, just a little two-centimeter black and blue star on my arm about six inches below my armpit." "Does it hurt?" He asked. "No." "It's pretty unlikely there's a clot there. It doesn't sound like phlebitis, and you have no history of it. You're already taking an aspirin a day for your arrhythmias, and since the aspirin serves as an anticoagulant, the likelihood of a clot for you is exceedingly low." I felt somewhat reassured but continued my questioning: "But why would I have a little lump?" "Those are very common. You probably have a lymph node that caught some microbe and swelled a bit. Don't worry about it." "Okay," I said, relieved. "But if it's still there when you get back in two weeks," Michael cautioned, "come in and see me." So I forgot about my black and blue star and my puffy BB, packed my suitcase, loaded about twenty-five pounds of books and overhead slides into my backpack along with my laptop, and headed for class.

After my class, Terry and I made a mad dash to the airport, and soon we were off to Geneva. The flight was smooth, and we even got five or six hours of sleep, which would come in handy in sustaining us through the intense three-day pre-plenary meeting we would soon attend. We stopped in Frankfurt to switch planes, and we deliberately sat on the left-hand side of the jet so we could enjoy the view of Lake Geneva and the spectacular backdrop of Mont Blanc and the Alps—if the clouds permitted. We weren't disappointed, and it was a marvelous short flight across a relatively cloudless Switzerland.

Asking the "What If" Questions

The pre-plenary meeting took place in the modernistic World Meteorological Organization building in Geneva, across the street from the Geneva office of the United Nations, the venue for the upcoming plenary. We met up with our colleagues—scientists, economists, and governmental agency leaders from around the world—who, along with us, made up Working Group II of the IPCC. As Working Group II, our responsibility was not to forecast how the climate would change as a result of the human dumping of waste products into the atmosphere—that is the job of Working Group I—but rather to ponder the question "So what if the climate changes? How will society and nature cope?" Of course, such straightforward, attention-focusing questions would never be allowed to headline a UN-sponsored report, so we went by the more staid name of "Working Group II: Impacts, Adaptation, and Vulnerability." Our goal in the pre-plenary session was to revise the Summary for Policymakers of our draft IPCC Assessment Report, which discussed how the world's people, rivers, crops, glaciers, plants, and animals would be affected by and forced to adapt to climate change and summarized suggested policies for helping them make the adjustment. (As scientists, we never recommend *which* policies should be chosen, as that is "policy prescriptive" and is the responsibility of the decision-makers who would be attending the plenary.)

The main friction during this pre-plenary meeting resulted from disagreements between climatologists and economists over the potential seriousness of global warming. Most climatologists in attendance believed that one cannot judge the extent of the damages that climate change could impose on nature and society simply by considering how climate change would affect things traded in markets and other items that were easily quantifiable in monetary terms (such as changed crop and forest yields and property loss due to rising sea levels). In my work with the IPCC, I wanted to value lost biodiversity and the heritage sites that would be destroyed if small island states like the Maldives and Tuvalu were flooded by rising sea levels. In general, I feel we should take a preventive approach to climate change, reducing greenhouse gas emissions now to lower the risk of serious dangers that climate change may pose later.

Some economists, however, note that small island states represent only a tiny fraction of the world's gross domestic product (GDP), and thus their demise would have almost no impact on the global economy when considered on a "one dollar, one vote" basis. They are reluctant to assign value to anything not traded in markets and tend to disagree with the idea of using a precautionary approach (e.g., cutting emissions now), contending that standard economic models show that spending significant amounts now to reduce emissions is not cost-effective, given that most of the benefits would only be felt far into the future. These economic analyses are misleading, however, since they do not tell the whole story.

Type I and Type II Errors

The decision on whether or not to act on many issues, climate change and medical situations included, often depends on what kind of error is of most concern. In climate change, if governments were to resort to the precautionary principle and act now, but their worries about climate change later proved to be unfounded and greenhouse gas emissions didn't greatly modify the climate, they would have committed what is known as a type I error. If governments took no hedging actions because of the uncertainty surrounding climate change issues, but then drastic climate change *did* occur, they would have committed a type II error. When debating with the economists at the meeting about climate change, I said that I'd rather risk a type I error. Later, when I had to make decisions about treatment for my lymphoma, I came to the same conclusion (see chapter 9).

Despite the disagreements within our group, we tried to bury the hatchet and focus on the deeper conflicts that were sure to surface at the plenary: the fierce battles waged by certain representatives who would try to bring the report in line with their countries' interests, even if it meant ignoring hard scientific evidence on global warming. Many of the debates would inevitably be the result of, or at least be blamed on, ambiguity regarding whether human-induced climate change was actually occurring and how severely global warming would affect the world during the next century or two. "Deep uncertainty" is the jargon I apply to situations in which both the probabilities of specified outcomes and their consequences are not well established. Climate change definitely qualifies, as does the treatment of many dread diseases.

The problem with having such a wide range of possible future climate change scenarios is that each special interest group can latch on to the outcome that best suits its position regardless of how likely or unlikely that outcome might be. Deep ecology groups risk type I errors, citing the most pessimistic outcomes, warning of catastrophe, and pushing for the implementation of energy taxes and other abatement policies as well as growth in renewable energy. The auto, oil, and other fossil fuel–intensive business groups, uncoincidentally, tend to be the extreme optimists in the global warming debate. They ignore the potential hazards of climate change, picking the least serious potential outcomes and stating that the uncertainties are still too large to enact climate policy, instead electing to risk type II errors. The media then dutifully report these dueling positions, further confusing the public with an endless stream of op-eds and stories quoting those who suggest that global warming is either "good for the Earth" or "the end of the world"—the two lowest-probability cases, in my view.

So it is the job of the IPCC and other groups to try to distinguish science from spin and make people aware of the usually very small probabilities of the most publicized, polarized outcomes. That's what we set out to do at the IPCC meeting in Geneva: We had to explain to the delegates the likely and not-so-likely ranges of possible outcomes caused by climate change, the nature of the deep uncertainties surrounding the climate problem, and the fact that both the probabilities and the consequences we outlined contained an uncomfortable element of ambiguity.

When Theory and Data Diverge

One of the problems in presenting climate change information, which we'll see again in looking at medical research, relates to the doctrine of "falsification." In order to test a theory, scientists typically perform an experiment that can provide results supportive of or contrary to their hypothesis. If the data are consistent with the hypothesis, the scientist holds on to the theory. If a hypothesis can't be falsified—that is, proven false—with contradictory data, the scientist continues to believe it but also continues to test it. As soon as the data collected from testing disagree with the hypothesis, the theory is "falsified" and must be rejected.

In reality, this falsification method can be fraught with errors because very often the data themselves are misgathered, the instruments and measurements are insufficient or inaccurate, or there are other, intervening factors that explain the divergence between data and theory. The theory may not be wrong, but just partial. These complexities not only frustrate scientists but also make policy decisions very difficult, since they may have to be made on the basis of partially tested theories. In the end, it is rare for some new observation or experiment to overthrow a theory or lead to a declaration that it is fully valid.

Theorists and Frequentists

In every course I teach, I like to demonstrate the difference between two ways of thinking by using the example of a coin toss. I flip a coin onto the back of my hand and cover it. "What is the probability that the coin under my hand is heads?" I ask my audience. "One-half," someone always shouts out. "How do you know?" I ask. "Well, the coin has two sides," is the typical answer. "You're a theorist! Now suppose you didn't understand the coin toss theory and didn't realize that there was an equal chance of flipping heads or tails. Could you still figure out the probability of flipping heads or tails?" "Well, yes, of course!" some student shouts out. "You just keep flipping it and count the number of heads and tails." "You're a frequentist! You want to put together a frequency chart. That is, you want to make a table with a column for heads and a column for tails, and then you want to flip the coin multiple times, put a mark in the appropriate column for each coin flip, and tally your results. If you flip it often enough and the coin is unloaded, you'll end up with frequency statistics showing an approximately 50 percent chance of flipping heads or flipping tails."

That is how scientists like to work: They like to have masses of data they can use to create probability distributions that depict the likelihoods of potential outcomes. If frequency distributions can be used, then scientists can make estimates that have high confidence levels. It's the same in medicine: Doctors like looking at data from clinical trials performed on hundreds of patients over many years, which can provide clear evidence as to whether certain treatments are effective, on average. Such frequentist logic is a useful, legitimate, and classical way of doing science.

Unfortunately, the questions associated with global warming, as well as many medical problems, can't be solved using falsification or frequency data, because they involve many components of deep uncertainty. In the case of global warming, much of the uncertainty relates to our incomplete knowledge of the role of clouds in global warming—do they contribute to it or lessen the effects?—and from our inability to foresee the state of the world in, say, 2100. What will the population be? What standard of living will people demand? Will they still be using Victorian industrial energy sources like coal, oil, and gas? Or will they have transitioned to renewable sources, such as solar or wind energy, or even safe and affordable next-generation nuclear energy? How can we know anything for sure about the future?

Such great uncertainty makes scientists *very* uncomfortable, as it makes accurate risk assessment difficult. When determining risk, scientists use the formula: risk = probability × consequence. But if deep uncertainty exists, and confident probabilities and consequences of events are themselves not well known, then how is a scientist to calculate risk? In other words, what do we do when a problem is important, frequency data on it are speculative, incomplete, or don't exist, and nearly every aspect of the problem is veiled by deep uncertainty? This is a question that scientists, from climatologists to medical doctors, must ask themselves constantly. Just as there are no data available on future global warming, in medicine doctors can't compile frequency data on rare diseases that have not been studied in clinical trials or on medical procedures that have not been done before or that have been performed only a handful of times.[2]

So what are both these groups of scientists to do? Should they refuse to think about these problems until frequency data are available, or should they use any and all other methods available to try to obtain a well-educated estimate of the likelihood of outcomes in the absence of adequate direct empirical testing? A patient with a rare disease is likely to urge his doctor to do the latter—and that is also the technique we had to sell to the delegates at the IPCC meeting.

Subjective Probabilistic Analysis

At the meeting, all our examinations of the future were based on a method called *subjective probabilistic analysis*, not on classical scientific falsification or frequentist logic. In this context, "subjective" means being based on knowledge, experience, intuitive judgment, and/or expertise, and *not* primarily on preexisting hard data, as too little exist in most situations in which subjective analysis is most useful.

This method can help us in climatology, medicine, and other disciplines in which problems lacking sufficient frequency data arise. Let's return to our coin toss example. Suppose there was going to be a $1 million bet on the outcome of the coin flip. Suppose also, as I often propose to my students, that one of the contestants involved was seen fooling around with the coin prior to the toss. "Do you think the probability of flipping heads is still one-half?" I ask the class. They giggle. "Well, probably not." Then I say, "But we don't have any frequency data to prove it since we haven't flipped it. How do you know that the coin is now likely to be unfair?" "A contestant who had a stake in the outcome was seen fooling around with it," a student replies. "Right," I said, "so we *do* have data; it's just not direct frequency data. It's data about the *process*."

This is where subjective probabilistic analysis, or "Bayesian updating"—named after Thomas Bayes (1702–1761), a clergyman who invented this method for assessing conditional probabilities—comes into play. A Bayesian, someone who uses subjective probability analysis, would probably think this way: The coin was unloaded to begin with, so the probability of flipping heads or tails was 50 percent each. That assumption is called a "prior probability"; it represents the Bayesian's belief, based on all the information available—luckily, in this case, frequency testing—to estimate the probability. But now we have new information—the fact that the coin was being handled and the handler had a stake in the outcome—and although it's not frequency data, we can still use it to modify our prior assumption and form a "revised prior"—what the Bayesian statisticians call an "a posteriori" probability, or simply an updated probability based on new information. We don't have precise sets of numerical data on the possibly altered coin, but knowing that it could have been tampered with in some way revises our prior belief that there was an equal chance of heads or tails.[3]

Nearly all of us use the Bayesian approach in our day-to-day lives to revise our beliefs about the likelihood of many events; in fact, a good portion of the human thought process is guided by Bayesian updating. Yet this method is still controversial in science. Some scientists, including many medical doctors, still seem to be living in the nineteenth century in this respect, thinking that for any question, infinite sets of replicable experiments should be performed, providing them with data from which they can calculate probabilities, assign accurate risk estimates, and "scientifically" tackle the problem at hand. Unfortunately, in the real world, as topics of inquiry become increasingly complex and involve questions about the future, scientists do not always enjoy the luxury of extensive, comprehensive, and reliable frequency data when they need them.

Assessing Risk

In climate change science, subjective probabilistic analysis is growing in importance; it has played a key role in recent developments, despite the grumblings of some old-fashioned frequentists. At the

1992 UN Conference on Environment and Development in Rio de Janeiro, for example, the governments of the world asked the IPCC to go head-to-head with the uncertainty surrounding global warming when they called for an international treaty to "prevent dangerous anthropogenic interference with the climate system" (which basically means to prevent the changes humans make to the atmosphere from causing severe harm).[4] They didn't define what they meant by "dangerous," leaving that to climatologists, economists, ethicists, and other policy analysts. We are scientists, however, and what is "dangerous" is a value judgment that should be made by governments. It is the policymakers who need to decide whether risks are acceptable or require new policies, or should be ignored or dealt with through adaptation. But we scientists can provide policymakers with information on which they can better make these decisions. In a medical setting, the science comes from medical research studies and doctors' opinions based on their experience with, data on, and knowledge of the subject. The "policymakers" are the patients, who, working together with their doctors, must make value judgments about what health risks to take.

Despite the uncertainties, there are some things that scientists know for certain, or at least with a high degree of confidence. Climate scientists know with a very high level of confidence, mostly from direct observations, that there is 30 percent more carbon dioxide and 150 percent more methane in the atmosphere now compared with 200 years ago—before the Industrial Revolution took off. These increases are a result of the growing number of people in the world and their demand for economic growth and higher standards of living, which have led to deforestation and the burning of coal, oil, and gas for energy. We also know with high confidence that carbon dioxide and methane trap heat near the Earth's surface. From that information, we can deduce that the more rapidly we dump our wastes into the atmosphere, the more pressure we will put on the system and the higher the probability that abrupt and catastrophic climatic "surprises" could be triggered.

Climate scientists can also study historical data to determine the relative rates at which new technologies were invented, how much investment it took to develop those new technologies, and how the prices of new energy systems dropped over time. These trends are referred to as learning curves. Our predictions about the future state of the world are also aided by computer models that have been proven to account accurately for some historical climate phenomena. The better our models explain the past, the more confidence we have that our processes are correctly incorporated in them and that they are likely to give us reasonable answers about the future.

However, in climate science, as in other fields—like medicine—the great amounts of uncertainty allow for potential consequences to range from the mild to the catastrophic. Whether it will be one degree Celsius or six degrees Celsius warmer in 2100—roughly the range that the IPCC assessment suggested was plausible—could be the difference between relatively mild change and devastating change. Thus, all that we scientists could do was describe a spectrum of possible outcomes and their approximate odds and assign confidence levels to our probability judgments—which were often no more than medium and sometimes even low. Then we could explain to the world community what aspects of the problem were well established and enjoyed a strong consensus despite some newspaper op-eds, politicians' statements, and oil company advertisements to the contrary, what aspects were supported by some evidence but could not be assigned high confidence, and what other components of the issue were highly speculative. In this way, when we discuss future climate change scenarios and consequences and assign probabilities and confidences to them, while they're not based on direct frequency charts, they *are* based on a large amount of credible empirical information and testing from past and present data.

This process is not unique to climate science. When a physician changes a patient's prescription because side effects emerge or decides to pursue a nonstandard treatment plan when the patient doesn't react favorably to the standard one, he or she is also using "Bayesian updating." In all fields of science, those of us who call ourselves "rationalists" would rather educate people using the well-thought-out, consistent, subjective estimates from all relevant and knowledgeable experts. Following Bayesian procedures will likely allow scientists, be they climatologists or medical doctors, to make more accurate judgments about probabilities and consequences than they could if they relied on completely unstructured inferences. Operating within a framework like Bayesian updating when confronting decision-making in the presence of uncertainty may help scientists avoid unnecessary cognitive errors.

Back to Geneva

The actual plenary meeting was finally gaveled to a start, and the first and most controversial issue on the agenda was Terry's work. Terry explained that after analyzing the behavior of some 1,000 species of plants and animals all around the world (as reported in the 150 papers that were used to perform the analysis), she and her team were able to show that about 80 percent of the species that exhibited some kind of meaningful change over the past forty years had changed in the direction that would be expected with warming—that is, trees flowered earlier, birds migrated to their breeding grounds sooner or laid their eggs earlier, and butterflies moved up mountains or to cooler regions closer to the poles. Thus, Terry declared, there was indeed a "discernible impact" of recent temperature trends on plants and animals.[5] This was a spectacular conclusion, for the Earth has "only" warmed up by about one degree Fahrenheit (0.6 degrees Celsius) in the past century, and most analysts simply assumed that it would be impossible to detect a correlation between such a "small" amount of warming and the behavior of plants and animals. But the worldwide data used in the statistical analysis showed a clear association.

In spite of the hard data supporting Terry's report, her findings were controversial because they were new and surprising, and they had the potential for political influence, since people around the world care deeply about plants and animals. Loss of biodiversity is often more "real" to people than some of the other effects of global warming. Thus, some of those at the IPCC meeting who opposed stringent climate policies wanted to do everything possible to minimize the importance of Terry's findings.

Terry and I were on the "witness stand" backing up this research for eight hours stretched over two days of the plenary. Despite our efforts to clearly explain the data, some delegates were quite nasty. The Saudi Arabians in attendance refused at first to agree to any language suggesting a clear scientific link between global warming and the movements of plants and animals, and many others followed suit.

We'd reached a stalemate, which was not encouraging, considering that in the United Nations most reports must be approved by a "consensus." By "consensus," the UN does not mean that *most* should agree but rather that *all* should agree. So, as is the practice, a "contact group," consisting of a selected group of the disagreers, a few neutral delegates, and the relevant lead authors (Terry and me, in this case) was formed. The goal of our group was to hammer out acceptable language on these findings for the report.

In the contact group, we haggled face-to-face over various concepts and wording until, in the wee hours of the morning, we were eventually able to formulate compromise language. Our two paragraphs of text conveyed the clear evidence that temperature trends were having an impact on plant and animal communities and included explicit statements on the lower level of confidence we had about how much of the observed response of plants and animals to local temperature trends of the past few decades could be linked to human-induced global warming. We could claim with high confidence that the behaviors and movements of plants and animals were due to observed climate change, but whether that change was due to human activities—"anthropogenic change"— would require considerably more sophisticated analysis (which Terry has recently completed and which indicates that humans are at least partly responsible for the observed changes to species).

Terry and I stumbled into our Geneva apartment around 3:00 a.m. after the contact group meeting, thrilled that we had agreed on language for our section and pleased that Terry's primary finding that recent temperature trends had affected plants and animals was still largely intact despite a number of weakening caveats in the compromise language. We were exhausted but ready to continue the battle. I never expected at that moment that this fighting mode would become routine for much of the next year and a half and that the future battles would be for my life.

Early the next morning, we dragged our sleep-deprived selves back to the UN building, where the computerized text of the entire IPCC document was projected onto large screens on two opposite walls. Our task that day was to review the Summary for Policy Makers and reach consensus on the text. The computer operator could track in red all the changes that were made to the text, so we could all see the proposed changes on the document projected on the walls. Delegates would raise their hands if they had objections and would propose modifications, which would also be input and tracked in red on the screen. Sometimes a single paragraph would take hours of painstaking negotiations.

At 9:00 a.m. on the third day of the plenary meeting, our contact group's two paragraphs, which had taken two days to negotiate, were flashed onto the screens. I waited with held breath to see who would complain first and whether the text would eventually be approved. The chairperson looked around, called for comments, and quickly said, "Seeing none." He slammed his gavel down on the table and accepted the text. I could feel the adrenaline draining from my system; I had been ready for a big fight, and after all that, it ended with a whimper—but that sure beat losing.

While I was heartened by this initial victory for sound science, we were still faced with a serious problem: Two days of the plenary had been spent finagling over the first major conclusion in the IPCC document, and we still had four or five more conclusions to cover. Only three days remained, and the delegates would go home at the end of the fifth day whether the document was approved or not.

But luck was on our side, and we got back on schedule. On the morning of the last day of the conference, I hopped into the shower, feeling elated that, after three years of work, we were actually going to achieve our final goal. Then, as my left hand applied soap to my right arm, there it was: a little bit of puffiness, just like when I had left California a week and a half earlier.

The puffiness was quickly forgotten and Terry and I rushed off to the last day of the meeting. Unfortunately, the Russians, Saudi Arabians, Chinese, and a few others seemed to have saved all their complaints for the last day. They made objection after objection to topics that didn't strike me as particularly controversial. Before we knew it, it was 11:00 p.m., and the document wasn't finished. The meeting was set to end at midnight, at which point the translators were free to go, as was stipulated in their contracts. Had these delegates intended all along to kill the document at the eleventh hour?

Robert Watson, the head of the IPCC, left the podium and was seen negotiating quietly but feverishly with the defiant delegations. Under Bob's strong leadership, the delegates slowly negotiated changes and accepted the modified text, but by that time the witching hour was ten minutes away, and there were still two paragraphs left to approve. Were we going to make it? At two minutes to midnight, the Russian delegate interrupted with yet more inexplicable complaints and requests for trivial changes. Other countries objected to the Russians' requests. We were going to fail. Was all this work for nothing?

But then Bob saved the day for the second time. He looked up and said, "Translators, three years' worth of work is on the line. Can you please stay two more hours and let us complete this document?" He knew that two or three delegations—the very same delegations who were completely capable of understanding English in the contact groups—had in the past refused to let the meeting proceed once the translators left, claiming it was a violation of procedure. The translators agreed to stay, but at 2:00 a.m. they'd had enough. We still had a few sentences left. Finally, the Russian delegate said, "I am putting this meeting under protest, but I will allow it to continue without translation." A Chinese delegate gave a five-minute speech in Chinese (for which no translation was available) to prove his point. Amazingly enough, after all that consternation, in a matter of fifteen minutes, the document was agreed upon, gaveled, and closed. A dog-tired, stressed-out group of scientists and delegates dragged themselves out of the UN building at 3:15 a.m. with a completed and approved text.

3 Whew! The Tests Are Negative, and I've Got a Plane to Catch

AFTER A FEW DAYS in the mountains of Switzerland trying to unwind after the incredible three-year process of producing the IPCC report, Terry and I flew home, where, recovering from jet lag, we had to face thousands of new e-mails and dozens of appointments with students eager to see their professors, who'd been gone for two weeks in the middle of the term.

I also had to face that same old slightly swollen underarm. A day after we returned home, my right arm got its usual soap-up in the shower, and I could tell that the puffiness and the BB were clearly still there. Before Terry even had a chance to badger me about it, I called Dr. Jacobs's office. "Ask Michael if he wants to see me," I told the nurse practitioner. "The lump is still there." An hour later, the nurse called back with an appointment time, and the next day, I went in.

Mike Jacobs was head of the section of primary care internal medicine at Stanford University Medical Center for a number of years while simultaneously serving as a professor and a clinician. He routinely makes the list of the top 100 doctors in the San Francisco Bay Area. Michael's patients include many Stanford docs, which is a sign of his excellence, much as a foreign food restaurant is deemed authentic when people of that ethnicity commonly patronize it. After too many frustrations with bureaucracies—especially HMOs—Michael set up a take-no-insurance private practice. This is apparently a major trend for fed-up doctors who want to maximize patient care but often can't manage to get the procedures and protocols they wish to perform through the hoops set up by cost-obsessed, nonphysician watchdogs. These problems occur both in nonprofit hospitals and in the for-profit medical insurance institutions with which most of us are forced to negotiate—although 40 to 50 million Americans can't even afford that service.

"It's probably just a swollen lymph node from some bug," Michael said, "but since you've had it for several weeks, why don't we do some tests?" "What are you looking for?" I asked. "Nothing," he said. "I just want to confirm that it's nothing." "What's the worst possible scenario?" I asked. He glanced at me, but even if he had been worried, he didn't show it. "Don't think about that; the probability of the worst-case scenario is low. These things are usually nothing." So I got orders for a chest X-ray and a blood test that would screen for enzymes that he said would help tell us "what it wasn't." I presumed the enzymes were associated with cancer, but nobody mentioned it.

I went in for the tests, and about three days later, the phone rang. Michael's news calmed me tremendously: "Everything is negative. I'm happy to report that your blood work and chest X-ray were completely normal." "That's great news," I said, "because I'm leaving on a one-month trip to Australia next week." I wanted to be in tip-top shape for a packed trip, including a meeting with the Australian Parliament, five talks on climate change, and, more important, a week's worth of vacation with Terry in southwest Australia, where we'd be looking for bird species we'd never seen. "Go and have fun," said Michael, "but if that lump is still there when you get back, I want to see you."

Later that day, I went to teach my climate change policy seminar. The class was fun. I can't wait for those kids to become our leaders; it's uplifting to see their fresh views and values and their insistence that our development activities be sustainable and fair. Fortunately for the world, they don't possess the standard careerism and greed that I see in Washington and so many other capital cities. *I just hope they remain determined*, I thought to myself, and I genuinely believe they will, based on the visits and e-mails and phone calls I've received from former students over the past few decades who still work on the fundamental principle that it is our job to make the world a better place than we found it.

The Land of Oz

The better place that was dominating my thoughts at that moment was Australia. Terry and I love going there—to Oz, as many affectionately call it, mimicking the local pronunciation: "Ozstraaaliah." As scientists and conservationists, Terry and I also took more than a passing interest in Australia's efforts to address the global warming problem. Although there were many Australians who wanted their country to join the Kyoto Protocol,[1] which would legally bind the country to meet certain greenhouse gas emissions targets, Australian Prime Minister John Howard, like the U.S. Congress and later the administration of George W. Bush, had strongly opposed the Kyoto Protocol on the grounds that it was "unfair" that countries such as the United States, Australia, and the western European nations were the only ones who were assigned binding emissions targets. Developing nations, such as China, India, and Indonesia, were "off the hook."

The Australian government as a whole was divided on the Kyoto Protocol, because Australia is a major coal producer and consumer and is the world's largest coal exporter. In 2000, coal met 85 percent of Australia's electricity needs and 40 percent of its overall energy needs, and it accounted for about 10 percent of its export merchandise trade.[2] However, very few Australian politicians honestly admitted that their hesitancy to sign on to the Kyoto Protocol or to enact other emissions reduction policies was related to their fear of lost income to special interests like the coal industry—and thus political pressure from these groups. John Howard's administration, like many others around the world, including our own here in the United States, used the much-favored excuse that there are just too many uncertainties in the science of global warming. But, as we've seen, on this issue, in medicine, and in many other fields, refusing to act in the face of uncertainty can expose us to considerable risks.

The Precautionary Principle

Not even the environmentally unfriendly John Howard could put a damper on our excitement about going to Australia. We began our trip in Sydney, where we stayed at the Harbourside Apartments on the recommendation of Paul and Anne Ehrlich, friends and colleagues in Stanford's biology department who were avid fans of Australia. If you've seen the movie *Crocodile Dundee*, you know approximately where the Harbourside Apartments are. Think back to the first scene, when the American reporter is sitting in Sydney against a backdrop of the harbor, the Harbour Bridge, and the opera house in the background. That's the view from the Harbourside Apartments. We arrived there at dusk, and when I looked out the window, there was a fireworks display just beginning over the bridge. "Terry, come here. Look at the fireworks they've put on to celebrate our arrival!" For the next twenty minutes, which I'll long remember, we watched the spectacular show in awe.

After a few days' vacation, we flew to Canberra to meet with the government's Greenhouse Office and some colleagues at the Australian National University. Terry gave a talk to government officials and university scientists on the work she'd done for the IPCC, and I spoke on how the media and political debates over global warming were distorting the nature of the actual science behind it. Then we had a dinner with several senators and members of Parliament in the Committee on Treaties who were debating whether Australia should sign the Kyoto Protocol.

The message we were there to convey was made more difficult because Richard Lindzen, a professor at Massachusetts Institute of Technology (MIT) with whom I have been disagreeing in intense public and private debates about the climate change problem for the past thirty years, had beaten us to Australia. He had convinced the Committee on Treaties that the science behind global warming was too uncertain to warrant taking action. It was our job to convince them that uncertainties in the science were inevitable but did not preclude an uncomfortable chance of dangerous outcomes and were no excuse for following a wait-and-see policy. I told the committee members that I could provide them with a range of outcomes that scientists thought to be plausible and could assign subjective probabilities to each outcome, but it was they who needed to make the value judgment about whether the risk of catastrophic outcomes was high enough to justify investing present resources as a hedge. I suggested that with the potential irreversibilities associated with global warming, this was the kind of problem that needed to be dealt with by doing research, forming tentative conclusions, and enacting policies based on them. I proposed that we needed to reevaluate the state of the world and our previous assessments every five years—the time span between IPCC reports—and crank up the controls if the science continued to suggest the potential for seriousness or crank them down if it appeared that we had overestimated the severity of the climate change problem. In short, my argument was "do a little, but learn a lot—and then redo." By the end of our dinner, I think the Australian legislators were at least partially convinced, and it was gratifying to know that Terry and I had presented an effective argument that swayed the opinions of several of them away from Lindzen's contrarian views.

This idea of acting preemptively in the absence of complete proof of harm in order to prevent potential damage to human health and the environment, is known as the *precautionary principle*. The precautionary principle, if acted on, can help prevent type II errors, the type to which policymakers and many others are typically averse. The precautionary principle is applicable not just to climate but to medicine and other subjects as well. In medicine, vaccinations are an excellent example of the precautionary principle; they are administered because there is a remote chance that the recipient could contract the disease the vaccine is meant to prevent, although in most cases, a type I error is committed—that is, the person never comes in contact with the disease, so the vaccine is never actually needed. An insurance premium never fully recovered by a claim of loss is another example of committing a type I error in order to avoid a type II error. Notice that in both examples, the serious risks are averted but are not cost free. A person must pay his or her insurance company a premium to obtain a policy, and the vaccine may have financial as well as health costs (e.g., the rare, but real chance of a bad reaction). As you will see throughout this book, I advocated the precautionary principle for the treatment of my disease multiple times, mainly in the form of preventive or maintenance therapy.

A Trip to Die For

The next week, our vacation began, and it remains vivid to me, especially in contrast to what lay ahead. We began in the Margaret River Valley, and after all the meetings we felt so alive in the mountains, by the ocean, admiring the beautiful parrots and other rare birds in the southwest corner of Australia, where the Indian Ocean meets the Southern Ocean and the large waves roll and crash into the rocky shore.

From the Margaret River Valley, we headed inland into the dry outback, the home of many a mallee fowl. The claim to fame of these ground-dwelling birds is that they build mounds on the ground that can measure about twenty feet wide and eight feet high, which they use as incubators for their eggs. The decomposition of the dead organic matter scratched up from the floor of the outback heats up the interiors of the mounds and keeps the mallee fowls' eggs warm. The birds never sit on their eggs at all; they let the mounds do the mothering for them. The male fowl, who tends the nest alone, is constantly exposing and covering the eggs, depending on their temperature. Some may call it laziness, but I think it's a stroke of evolutionary genius. I was very keen on seeing a mallee fowl.

One of our student guides had heard that the largest mallee fowl mound in that part of Australia was located near where we'd been driving, in the middle of a thicket of mallee bushes. He had been given the coordinates of the megamound by another student who had studied it and planned to use his global positioning system (GPS) as our "compass," so we followed him into the brush. A half an hour and ten or fifteen nicks and scratches into our trek, the GPS told us that we were within 300 feet of the mound. Finally, through a thick maze of branches, we saw an incredible sight: a five-foot-high, twenty-foot-wide mound of dirt and litter right in the middle of a small clearing. It was the kind of thing Hollywood would turn into a film about an extraterrestrial invasion, but in fact these were very terrestrial creatures, these ground birds, and their works of architecture were truly amazing.

We didn't walk on the mound because we didn't want to damage it in case there were eggs in it, but we circumnavigated it and climbed up in the trees to look down on it. No mallee fowl in sight, however. While the students and I had been poking around, Terry separated herself from the group and was down on her knees peering into the brush. "Come over here!" She suddenly whispered, and everybody headed her way. We looked past about twenty tree trunks and lots of scrub, and there, walking along the ground, was the mallee fowl! We sat very still, and in about five minutes, it came within ten feet of us on its way back to the mound but then scurried away very unhappily when it saw us. "Time to go," Terry said. "It *does* need to tend the nest."

Later that night, we returned to Albany and sat down to a wonderful meal in the Albany Hotel, replete with some excellent Margaret River wines. I couldn't get the mallee mound out of my mind. It was such a spectacular piece of nature, and it was yet another reason why I did not want the world to warm up four to ten more degrees Fahrenheit (some two to six degrees Celsius). Warming of this magnitude would push many creatures hundreds, if not thousands, of kilometers out of normal range, forcing them to cross hostile habitats to try to find suitable locations, which could disappear altogether if climate change is rapid. Nevertheless, after a great steak and a fabulous red wine, I couldn't help but feel content.

Terry and I went upstairs, and I hopped in the shower again. Unfortunately, the mound that struck me this time was not that of the mallee fowl, but that persistent bump in my armpit. I thought it had disappeared, but once again, there it was.

—|⊢—

My first destination on arriving home was Dr. Jacobs's office. "What do you think, Michael?" I asked. "We'd better do more tests," he said. So I snapped out of vacation la-la land and went back to the Stanford University Medical Center. I went through another ghouling and then paid a visit to the ultrasound technician, who forcefully pushed his probe into my little puffy spot. It was pretty uncomfortable, but the results were worth the pain. The blood test came back negative again, and the ultrasound merely showed an unsuspicious enlarged lymph node. Everything was essentially normal. I was phenomenally relieved, more in finding out that I wouldn't have to miss a long-scheduled trip with the Ehrlichs and Tom Lovejoy[3] to Venezuela, Ecuador, and the Galapagos Islands than in finding out that I wasn't suffering from any sort of nasty illness. After all, nearly every medical scare I had faced in the previous fifty-six years had been resolved without much hassle, so why not this one too? But in reality, after going for three months with what was being called an "enlarged lymph node," I was starting to become concerned—and so was Michael.

During the next few weeks, there were a few times when I was in the shower and thought that my lump was completely gone, because the puffiness seemed to have disappeared. *Finally*, I thought to myself, *this swollen lymph node is no longer reacting to the bug it caught, and soon I won't even notice it*. But then I would poke deeper and realize that while the puffiness had gone down, the lump had not, and in fact, it felt a little *bigger*. I tried not to think about it, but I began to realize, even while snorkeling with penguins in the Galapagos, that there would soon be surgery in my life.

CHAPTER

4 | Taking My Lumps:
Biopsy Blues

AFTER MAKING THE CALL to Mike Jacobs that I'd been dreading, he called back to say, "I've made an appointment for you with my old friend Harry Oberhelman.[1] He's a wonderful surgeon. He'll do a biopsy on you, and then we'll see once and for all what this lump is. Four months is too long."

The next day, Terry and I went to Stanford Hospital and got to know Harry Oberhelman, perhaps better than I might have liked. Harry and his young resident poked and prodded me from top to bottom. "Oh yeah, there's your lump. Uhhhhh, well, it feels like you have one here on your groin, too," said the resident. "There are lumps in my groin area?" I asked, very unhappily. "Yeah," she said, "but swollen lymph nodes in the groin aren't rare. I wouldn't worry. We'll probably still only biopsy the one under your armpit; that one should give us all the information we need." (I was much less worried about multiple biopsies than about what multiple lumps meant!) Harry then went into the details of the biopsy surgery, and he said I'd need to take a few days to recover afterward.

"But why do I need surgery? Can't we just stick a needle into my lump and do the biopsy that way?" "I'm a surgeon. I don't do

42

that kind of thing," Harry said, "but I know people who do. I agree with your point; why should we do unnecessary surgery? Let me call the SWAT team." I wondered why I even had to ask about a nonsurgical biopsy but realized that the senior surgeon's job was doing surgery. I was sent to him for surgery, and he was just doing his job. I was impressed, however, that he was so cheerful and willing to accommodate my request. All I was trying to do was avoid getting cut up when I could "just" have a needle poked into my arm.

Half an hour later, the "SWAT team," consisting of a much younger doctor with an intern, a resident, and a medical student, arrived. Once again, I got the feel-up treatment from head to toe. This time, there were not two but *four* sets of hands studying my lumps, but I kept my cool. I knew I was in a teaching hospital, and the pros of being there (having the world's leading researchers studying my problems and having access to the top doctors in many fields) still far outweighed the cons (being prodded by neo-phytes and experiencing a total loss of privacy).

The "needle doctor" consulted with his crew: "We could get this. Let's use this one here," he said, pointing to what I thought was the same old lump in my arm. They discussed axillary this and centimeter that, and it all sounded like the procedure would be routine, but I was still not looking forward to it. Although I've al-ways been good with shots and other medical procedures, the thought of having a large-bore needle forced deep into my arm didn't sound quite as easy as going in for my annual flu shot.

"Are you going to use Novocain?" I asked. "No," the doctor said confidently. "Injecting the Novocain would hurt as much as the biopsy needle; it's not worth it." "Okay." That made me feel better.

Before he stuck me, the doctor felt my arm very carefully once again, and finally he said, "Okay, I got it." I looked over, and his fin-gers were not on my lump. "Wait a minute," I said. "That's not where the lump is; it's lower down." "I'm gonna stick this big one," he said, "which is deeper. You probably never even felt it." He was right. I looked at Terry, and we both knew the results could not possibly be good.

Your Results Are In

The next day, Terry and I had a plane to catch to New York, to visit my then–ninety-three-year-old dad, who was very excited about seeing us. I always tried to schedule a side trip to New York whenever Terry and I flew east, and since we had to go to Annapolis anyway to meet with Tom Lovejoy about the book we were writing together, we took the opportunity to drop in on my dad for a couple of days and had a great time. I thanked my lucky stars that I had thought of and was able to have the needle stick rather than the full biopsy surgery, which could have forced me to cancel the New York trip since I would have been laid up for a few days. Given my dad's age, I often had the uneasy feeling that every trip could mark the last time I would see him, so it was important to me to be there. In retrospect, I'm glad I made it out that time, because my next three scheduled trips to New York did not happen. Fortunately, there were sixteen trips after those three that did happen—right up to my dad's death at age ninety-seven in September 2004. My dad never did find out about my cancer, and we figured it was for the best, since it was the last thing a man nearing 100 needed to worry about.

From New York we took the train to Maryland, which was certainly easier than hassling with more airplanes. There we met with Tom Lovejoy, and the next day we flew home from Baltimore. I vividly remember the surreal scene that took place in the Baltimore airport. Terry boarded the plane about ten minutes before the gate was going to close, and I stayed behind because I wanted to call my office to find out if anything important had happened that I needed to know about. "Don't miss the plane!" Terry warned me, and she was right that there wasn't much time. I smiled at her and waited for my administrative assistant to answer my call. "Hi, Françoise, how are things going there?" She rattled off a list of phone calls that I had received, and toward the end, she mentioned, "Oh, by the way, Michael Jacobs called and gave me a number where you can reach him." "Michael Jacobs?" I asked incredulously. "Yeah, your doctor," she said, probably wondering if I was losing my mind. "You mean his *office* called?" "No, *he* called, and he left a private number and said that you should call him as soon as you had a chance."

Butterflies hit my stomach. In the ten years that I had been seeing Michael, he had *never* told me to call his private line ASAP. *Hopefully this is good news and he called me to tell me that*, I thought to myself, but the butterflies were getting stronger. With only five minutes before the gate would close, I called Mike back, hoping desperately that he would answer the phone. He did. "Hi, Steve. Your results are back, and I'm afraid they're not great." "What does that mean, Michael?" "Well, you have a non-Hodgkin's B-cell lymphoma." By that point, my butterflies were about to lift me off the ground. "What does that mean?" I asked. He said, "Well, fortunately, you have a B-cell and not a T-cell cancer.[2] B-cell cancers tend to be less severe, but you'll still need to start treatment right away. But don't panic, Steve. I want to assure you that Stanford is 'lympho-mecca.' It is the best hospital in the world for this kind of disease, and the oncologists here have many good treatments and very high success rates."

"I've scheduled an appointment for you with Harry Oberhelman tomorrow," Michael continued, "so that he can biopsy the lump." After all the work I'd done to get out of the biopsy surgery and have a needle biopsy instead, I can't say I was thrilled at the prospect. "Well, if you already know what I have, why do we need to do the surgery? Why don't I just get on with the chemo or whatever else I need to do?" I asked. "We'll need more tissue to know precisely how to type and stage you so that the best treatment plan can be designed. Don't worry, Steve; I'll call the head of the oncology department and get you the best lymphoma doctor this hospital has. You'll get through this." "I sure hope so, Michael." I hung up and thought, *The last thing I want to do is to miss my airplane and be stuck here any longer than I have to be.* I hurried to the gate and entered the plane with only seconds to spare.

One of our good friends, Diana Wall, was flying with us that day. She was sitting in the aisle directly across from us, and though I am quite fond of her, I wasn't in the mood for chit-chatting; I desperately needed some time to think. I did not want to discuss my recent diagnosis with anyone, because I didn't know anything about how severe it was or what I'd have to go through to get rid of it, and that itself was as big a stress as the diagnosis. I tried to put on a happy face when I walked into the airplane cabin, but Terry saw right through me. She looked at me gravely after I told her I'd talked to Mike Jacobs and asked, "How bad?" "B-cell lymphoma," I said quietly. She grasped my hand. "Oh God, we'll fight this together. We'll get through it," she said.

That was the weirdest airplane flight I've ever had. All the way home, I felt like my stomach was in my throat, like somebody had died. I thought about the prospect of dying myself, and it was so alien. I just had a few lumps, and I felt fine, but I knew that lymphoma was a life-threatening disease. I tormented myself by wondering whether my case was curable, how mild (or not) it was relative to others, what the treatments would do, what the prognosis was, what the monitoring techniques were for measuring progress, and what kind of hell I was going to have to go through to deal with it. I was frightened, but at the same time I was absolutely resolute that I was going to do whatever it took to beat the disease. Not only was I thinking about Terry and my dad and what this would do to them, but I was thinking of my kids, who were just emerging from adolescence and beginning to grow into exceptional individuals. The last thing they needed was to lose their father at this important stage in their lives. And then there was my work. We still needed all hands on deck for the fight against global warming, and I knew I could pull my weight in that arena. In fact, I remember thinking to myself, *Life isn't fair! My scientific bête noire, Richard Lindzen [the MIT anti–global warming scientist], smokes two packs a day; he won't outlive me!* I guess I needed all the inspiration I could get, so thanks, Dick, for that one. But even in the face of such motivation, I honestly didn't know whether maybe this time I had run out of luck. What was most frustrating, perhaps, was that sitting on a plane precluded me from researching my disease on the Web or elsewhere. I was literally flying blind with no relief for my left brain.

A "Good Idea"—But Not Yet Routine

The next day, both Terry and I had appointments at Stanford Hospital. First, we went to see Michael Jacobs, who told me that in two days Harry Oberhelman would take out one of my lumps; then the pathology lab would do a detailed analysis of it to determine which doctor and what treatments would be best for me. "How long will it take to get the results?" I wondered out loud. "About a week." "How quickly will I recover from the surgery?" "It won't take very long. Ask Harry." "I have to go to Colorado in four days," I said, "not only to attend a meeting that I've been looking forward to for a year, but to see my sister Liz and her whole family, who are meeting us there. They've already left San Diego and are headed to Colorado just to see us." "You can go to Colorado," Michael said, "but depending on what is found when the typing is done on the sample Harry takes, you might have to come home early."

Later that day, we went to see Terry's surgeon in the breast clinic. Terry had had biopsies before, none of which had found cancerous tissue, thankfully, but she was still diligent about going in for periodic checkups. "I always thought I was going to be the one with cancer," Terry said as we walked through the oncology wing for the second time that day, "not you." "Well, as long as I have it, you'd damn well better not," I said. She tried to smile, and we went to see the doc.

The appointment was supposed to be about Terry, whose exam went fine, to our great relief, but we ended up talking about me. When I told the surgeon that I was going to have a surgical biopsy in two days, she said, "When you get your biopsy, I think you should have *two* of your lymph nodes removed rather than one." "Why is that?" I asked. "Because the pathology lab will basically destroy the lymph node they use to type you, and then you won't have any other samples. I understand that Ron Levy's[3] lab is working on creating individualized treatments for people's specific strains of cancer, so it'd be a good idea to send a second lymph node there, where they'll freeze it and have it on hand in case Ron invents something." It sounded like pretty good advice to me.

The next day, I checked in for biopsy surgery at 8:00 a.m. I got my first IV, and I was really surprised at how little it hurt. I was still nervous, though, and the anesthesiologist sensed it and gave me a shot of Novocain, which I realized, in retrospect, hurt more than most IVs put in by nurses.

The anesthesiologist asked me, "How conscious do you want to be during the procedure? For these biopsies, we don't use general anesthesia." "Well, what were you planning on using?" I wanted to know. "Versed. It's a new drug made by Roche that allows you to be conscious throughout the procedure, though you won't re-member a thing." "You mean I'll be able to feel things?" I asked with horror. He said, "Well, not really, because we'll give you local anesthesia, too. How much do you want to be out of it? It's really your decision." "Is there anything that I need to do or move or de-scribe? Is there any way I can help by participating?" I asked. "Not at all," said the anesthesiologist. "Then beam me up, Scottie! Give me the maximum amount that isn't going to cause any side ef-fects." "This drug has no side effects. It operates by suppressing your central nervous system and making you forget, but you won't have any aftereffects once it wears off." "Hmmmm," I said. "Don't give it to me yet because I have to talk to Dr. Oberhelman when he arrives." So, the anesthesiologist gave me a mild sedative, which wasn't enough to knock me out.

Thinking Ahead

When Harry arrived, smiling, my head was still pretty clear. I told him what Terry's surgeon had said, and Harry said, "Yeah, I've heard about Ron Levy's work. That's a good idea. I'll take two samples today and I'll send the second one over to Ron. Thanks for telling me." Once again, a senior doctor was saying, "Good idea, patient. I'd be happy to do that." That was definitely not the experience I had later with all the physicians I encountered during my treatments. Also, once again, as I was to learn many times over, thinking ahead (about the second sample, in this case) would give me a leg up in fighting my cancer—how much so I couldn't have imagined at that stage. From that time forward, Terry and I made a point of asking many questions and always prepping before my appointments at the hospital so that we could cover all bases as best we could. I encourage all cancer patients, their friends, their family members, and their advocates to do the same.

The next thing I remember about the surgery was Harry looking at me, patting the big pad secured under my right arm and saying, "Everything went fine. I'm going to send one lump out for typing and the second over to Ron Levy's lab on the first floor of pathology, as you suggested. I checked with somebody about that and was told that sending a sample to Ron should be routine, but nobody had ever told me." What a lucky break that we had chatted with Terry's breast surgeon two days earlier! "By the way," I told Harry, "I thought you were using a *local* anesthesia, but I was totally out the whole time. I didn't feel a thing." "It *was* a local, and actually, you weren't completely knocked out. We just gave you Versed, so you don't remember anything." "That's as good as being out to me." "No," he said, "it's better because there are no side effects from this drug like there are from general anesthesia." I marveled at the wonders of modern medicine and hoped there were more miracles for my real problem, the lymphoma.

I let Harry know that I was leaving for Colorado in two days, and he said, "If you don't have any pain, swelling, or fever, it's okay with me. Just don't swim, don't lift anything with your right arm, try not to sweat, take it easy, and let your wife drive." "Yessir," I said. I joined Terry in the waiting room, and we went home.

"You Can't Fool Around with This"

We took a quick flight to Denver and then headed for the hills in a rental car. We were going to Leadville, a historic village nestled into the Rockies at 10,000 feet, where we would meet my sister, my brother-in-law Mike, and our nieces. I hadn't been able to talk to any of them because they'd been traveling, so I hadn't been able to tell them about my lymphoma. I did tell my brother Peter in New York, and I told him to relay the info to Liz if she called.

When we met Liz and Mike in Leadville, they'd already heard the news from Peter. They hadn't mentioned it to their kids, though, because they were afraid they might relay the information to their grandfather. Actually, I hadn't even told my *own* kids; I was planning on talking with Becca and Adam when we returned home. So we agreed that no kids would find out for another week.

We drove over Independence Pass at sunset and dropped down into Aspen, where Terry and I would be attending the Energy Modeling Forum, as we did almost every year. We had taken our nieces to Aspen with us quite a few times, and they told such wonderful stories about the good times we'd had that their mother decided she wanted to come along. We'd arranged this weeklong vacation, but I feared that it wasn't going to last a week, because as soon as that pathology report came in, I suspected I would be ordered to come home.

At the start of the Energy Modeling Forum, I warned the conference organizers that we might have to leave early. I told them a carefully formulated half-truth: I had a long-standing medical problem involving arrhythmias, and my doctor, who was about to go on sabbatical, could only see me later that week. I made it clear that we wouldn't be able to stay for the entire conference, and I suggested that the organizers schedule my presentation for the first day of the forum, just in case. They looked at me quizzically, because I'd never mentioned the arrhythmias before. "And why would you go home to get a simple medical test from one doctor when there are plenty of doctors who could do it right here?" I realized it seemed somewhat far-fetched, but when the organizers saw that I wasn't going to budge, they dutifully rescheduled my talk to the first day of the meeting.

On that Monday morning, the phone rang. It was Michael Jacobs telling me that the pathology report had come in, they knew exactly what I had, and that he had found an excellent oncologist for me. The only problem was that she was about to head off to a two-week-long conference, so Mike had squeezed in an appointment for me to see her before she left, on Thursday of that same week. In fact, he told me that Thursday was not her usual day in clinic; she'd made an exception to see me. "What's her name?" I asked. "Sandra Horning." "Did you recommend her, Michael?" "I didn't, but I wish I could take credit for it," he said, "because the senior lymphoma doctor here said she's the best person in the world for treating what you have. When you see her Thursday, she'll explain all the details to you—the severity of your lymphoma, the treatments she recommends, and the timetable she envisions. I don't know much about cancer, but I *do* know you'll be in the best hands there are. Sandra and her team actually *invented* many of the elements of the treatment protocol that they'll probably use on you." "Any chance I can push the appointment back a week?" I asked, desperately wanting to spend more time with my sister and her family. "No, you can't fool around with this, Steve.

You need to come home and get your treatment started. Take another day in Colorado, and fly home Wednesday. You *need* to see Sandra on Thursday." "Will do," I said, disappointed.

I gave my talk at the conference and excused myself shortly thereafter. I explained my "circumstances," sticking to my original story, and apologized to everyone about having to leave on such short notice. "But it's nothing serious," I said, lying through my teeth. Given my ignorance of the disease, I just couldn't bring myself to tell colleagues at the Energy Modeling Forum about my lymphoma, even though many were my friends. I've done plenty of things in my life designed to turn heads, but that was not the way I wanted to get further attention, so I put on a happy face and headed out.

On my way out, I approached one of my colleagues, Lou Pitelka,[4] who had been diagnosed with chronic lymphocytic leukemia[5] many years earlier, and I asked him how he was. I couldn't help but be a little emotional; I was very sympathetic and told him how courageous he was for fighting the disease and not allowing it to get in the way of his work and other passions. Having figured out that my intense interest was more than just a polite gesture, he called me up a week later and asked, "What's wrong?" Over time, I learned from people like Lou that there's a community of cancer patients out there who offer each other mutual support, which has proven helpful in facing the disease, surviving treatment, and overcoming the horrors of the disease. But I didn't know any of that then.

Getting to the Bottom of It?

When Terry and I got home, the first thing we did was search the Web for information on Sandra Horning. We learned that two years earlier, Sandra had received a prize for being the best clinician at Stanford Hospital, and a year before that, she had been appointed full professor in oncology and bone marrow transplantation. "Well, this sure seems to be her specialty," Terry said. "Any woman who makes full professor by age fifty in that male-dominated bastion must be first-rate," I quipped. That turned out to be a very good assumption, or Bayesian prior.

Terry and I went to the Oncology Day Care Center the next day, and the room was jam-packed with people. Many of them were middle-aged women, most with breast cancer, we presumed. Some had big masks with pink filter disks, indicating that they were either sick or in the middle of chemotherapy treatment and were not supposed to breathe in germs. If I looked carefully enough, I could see that there were a lot of wigs in the room. Still, it was sometimes hard to tell who was the cancer victim and who was the spouse, the parent, the child, or the friend, as almost no one was there alone. I was glad to have Terry there by my side.

I was told that Dr. Horning had requested a blood sample from me, which immediately made me nervous. I steeled myself and walked into the ghouling room, where the nurses proceeded to extract quite a few vials' worth of my blood. They stuck them into a big plastic tube. "What are you doing with that tube?" I asked. "Oh, it's a pneumatic tube," the nurse said. "Your samples will be placed in this chamber and transported by a vacuum to the lab, which is at the far end of the building. We'll have the results back in an hour, in time for you to meet with the doctors." This was obviously a well-honed operation.

An hour or two later, I was called into an examination room. About half an hour after that, a young doctor and a medical student arrived. The doctor was a research Fellow, five years post-M.D., and an assistant to Sandra Horning. He listened to my story with interest, paying careful attention when I relayed that we'd already found another lump. "Oh, we're pretty good at feeling lumps," he said, "and I'm sure you have a lot more than the ones Harry's team found." He then examined me, saying, "Here's one, there's one, here's one, there's one," and so forth. I then let his hand guide mine over a few of the lumps, and it was clear that he was right. He found a particularly worrisome one in my neck, and as he pushed it around, I started to feel very queasy.

"So, what's the story?" I asked him, having already told him that I wanted to know everything about my disease and treatment so that we could plan a course of action together. He looked at me quizzically, as if he couldn't believe that I was going to insist on being involved in formulating my treatment, and then said gravely, "You have mantle cell lymphoma." "What's that?" Terry snapped. "And why do you sound so serious?" "Well, it's a pretty rare disease. Only about 5 percent of B-cell lymphomas are mantle cell, and we only have about eight or ten years' experience treating it in the United States and maybe two or three more in Europe, so there isn't a lot of information about it." "Well, is it indolent or aggressive?" I asked, having already read on the Web that lymphoma commonly comes in a slow-growing but hard-to-shake indolent form or a fast-growing, life-threatening, but easier-to-treat aggressive form. "Well, it's kind of like both." "Both?" "It's indolent *and* aggressive." "What do you mean?" "Well, when mantle cell lymphoma is in its growth phase, it spreads quickly, like an aggressive cancer, but it's also really hard to get rid of, like an indolent one." I said, "And you don't have much information?" "No." *So, the gods of irony have given me a research disease*, I thought to myself.

I continued my questioning: "Is it treatable?" "Oh yes, and not only is it treatable, but we have new protocols that are vastly more effective than the old ones and good enough data to suggest that we can successfully fight this." The Fellow stressed again, however, that because the disease was relatively rare, and therefore few patients had been monitored extensively, there was almost no frequency information available that we could use to determine the relative probabilities of success given various lengths, types, and intensities of treatments. They had historical data on a few dozen patients from which they were able to formulate the new-and-improved protocol that they planned to use on me, but that was all the information that was out there at the time.

"Don't worry," he said. "Dr. Horning will tell you everything right after your bone marrow biopsy." "Bone marrow biopsy?" "Yeah, we need a sample of your marrow in addition to the lymph node [extracted by Dr. Oberhelman] so that we can stage and type you in order to prescribe the best possible chemotherapy regimen for you. This cancer likes to hide in bone marrow, so that's where we can get the best read of it." "Will that require surgery?" "Oh no, we'll do it right here and now," he said. "It only takes a few minutes." "I presume this is not fun," I said, grimacing. "No, I can't say it's *fun*," he said, "but I'll give you a local anesthetic. It'll prevent you from feeling the initial entry of the needle. When it goes into your bone, you'll feel it, but not for very long." Terry walked over to me and grabbed my hand. "I'm here," she said. "We'll get through this."

The Fellow and the med student left and came back about five minutes later with a big package. I could hear them ripping open the kit that would be used for my bone marrow extraction, and I started to look over at it but decided that seeing the needle would not help me. I knew it was going to be far larger than anything I had been drilled with before, because it had to be strong enough to crack through my bone. "What bone will you take the sample from?" I asked. "Well, we take the sample out of the back of your hip." The Fellow moved my finger over the V-shaped indent in my rear hipbone. He said, "We like to insert the needle here because there's less of a chance of it skidding. It'll slide right in, and there's very good bone marrow fluid there."

The easygoing fourth-year medical student who was helping the Fellow sensed that I was in need of distraction, so he struck up a conversation. Terry and I learned that he already had a Ph.D. in biological science and was getting his medical degree because he wanted to do research *and* practice medicine. "Do you also have a Ph.D.?" I asked the Fellow. "Yup," he said. "Well," I said, "I guess it's consoling to know that I'll at least be getting drilled by two Ph.D.'s." The Fellow snickered and said, "Oh no, you'll want a *doctor* for this one." The joking put me a little more at ease, but the bone marrow extraction was still a spooky experience. I was injected with lidocaine, the local anesthetic, and it stung quite badly. The Fellow explained that it was because he had to stick the needle into the membrane (periosteum) around my hip bone in order to maximize the numbing effect. About five minutes later, as I was lying on my stomach with Terry insisting that I look at her and hold her hand, he unpackaged the needle and said, "You're going to feel this." It was the understatement of the year.

Once the needle was actually in, I felt only a dull ache. "We have to take an aspirate," the Fellow said. "What's that?" "It's a fluid sample. We have to suck it out. It's going to feel really weird, but it'll come out quickly." They attached what appeared to be a suction pump onto the needle and sucked out a few cubic centimeters (cc's) of fluid. "Weird" wasn't the word or feeling that came to mind; it was more along the lines of sharp, tingling pain dispersed along the bone.

Fortunately, the suctioning was over in about ten seconds. The needle was still in my back, though; I could feel the dull ache. "Now, we need a physical sample," the Fellow said. He had told me that while the aspirate wasn't usually too grueling, the physical sample would be. The aspirate had hurt like hell, so I didn't think his credibility was too high. But actually, obtaining the physical sample, which involved jamming the needle farther into my hip and taking out a piece of the inside of my bone, was less painful than anticipated. The problem came at what I thought was the end of the procedure, when the Fellow said, "You know, I don't think this sample is adequate." "What are you going to do?" I asked. "I'm going to give you another lidocaine shot and reinsert the needle in a different spot, about two inches away." My heart sank; I had been feeling victorious about surviving the extraction, and now I had to do it all over again. Was there going to be a third and a fourth time? I could feel my strength wavering.

The second time was no better than the first. At that point, as I was still lying helplessly on my stomach, Sandra Horning came in, looked at the samples, and said, "Those are fine. Send them to the lab." She and the Fellow patched up my back and told me to sit up slowly, and that it would hurt. It did, but they promised there would be no side effects other than the stiffness. There weren't any.

"Are You Sure You Want to Know Everything?"

I regained my composure and focused in on Sandra Horning. She was a petite, very cheerful, easy-mannered person. Sandra was a full professor, and so was I, and I made it clear at the outset that I didn't like titles. She said she didn't either, so we went on a first-name basis from then on. I introduced Terry and told Sandra that she was a biology professor at the University of Michigan, but she was going to be on sabbatical for the whole year to be with me.

Then we got down to business. I told Sandra my philosophy of decision analysis and emphasized that I wanted to learn absolutely everything about my disease, especially since it was rare and still a "research disease." I wanted to help assess how to weigh the probabilities and consequences of treatment options and pick the best possible combination to maximize my odds of survival. I'm sure this was not the usual introduction she or the Fellow got from new patients.

Sandra looked me straight in the eyes and said, "Are you sure you want to know everything?" "Yes," I said nervously. She then began to explain how mantle cell lymphoma was discovered, what data were available on it, what their standard protocol was for treating it, and what the chemotherapies were like. She stressed that before Stanford's new protocol had been implemented, 50 percent of her mantle cell lymphoma patients were dead within two years, and 90 percent didn't make it past the five-year mark. With the new protocol, however, she hadn't lost a patient in four years. Even though there were only a few dozen patients who had received the new treatment, her four-year, zero percent mortality record was clearly statistically significant.

I sat there on the examining table where I had just had my bone drilled into, looking into the face of this pleasant woman who was going to save my life, watching her lips move, and hearing her spoken words, but after a while I was completely overwhelmed, and I felt like I couldn't make any sense of it. I tried to snap out of it, telling myself, *You have got to listen to what she says. She's telling you about your disease. You need to know all this.* But my unconscious was saying, *No, you don't want to know all this.* I looked over at Terry. Her notebook was open, and she had already scribbled down a paragraph of notes. *I don't have to listen to this quite so carefully*, I said to myself. *I'll just pretend I'm listening. Terry will back me up on this one.* That's the first time I ever remember having an out-of-body experience. I was physically there, and I saw Sandra's lips moving and heard her voice resonating through the room, but the rest of me was somewhere else. It reminded me of that scene from the Spielberg movie *Saving Private Ryan* when the troops land at Omaha Beach and men are being machine-gunned down right and left. All of a sudden, the hero blanks out and everything goes into slow motion. Nothing seems real for about ten seconds, and then he snaps back to reality.

My slow-motion mode lasted for what must have been many minutes. I didn't even remember hearing that Sandra was a professor of medicine specializing in oncology and bone marrow transplantation, and that after all the chemo, she would reward me with a bone marrow transplant, something I didn't even think I needed at the time. (Later on, I realized I had been in utter denial about the bone marrow transplant. This experience helped me to be more sympathetic toward others who refused to acknowledge how serious their condition was and that certain grueling treatments would be necessary.)

Everyone Needs an Advocate Sometimes

Despite wanting to be an active participant in treating my cancer, this out-of-body experience reminded me that when dealing with a dread disease, at times an advocate is essential—even for the most rational of scientists. Having Terry's eyes, ears, and mind working at the same time mine were was valuable in itself, as it allowed me to bounce ideas off her later and helped us make better decisions about my treatment. But when my unconscious took over in an effort to protect me and I was unable to take in information about my condition, Terry was my lifeline, my sole source of information about what had happened. She would brief me afterward, when I was ready to hear the information, and she would comfort me as well. Through her, I learned that having an advocate is not a sign of weakness but an indication that the patient is using all resources available in the hopes of being restored to health.

I highly recommend that all patients try to get advocates. In choosing an advocate, you should decide what level of interaction with medical personnel fits your personality, knowledge base, and medical situation. Find an advocate who can intercede at the level you want and help you think ahead about questions you should ask and requests you should make. Of course, your advocate should be someone you trust with very personal information and feel comfortable interacting with, so friends and family members are often ideal. Perhaps your family doctor would even be up to the task; although I don't know of many examples of it, I suspect that if asked, personal physicians might well be willing to help. You may be hesitant to ask someone to perform such an enormous task for you, but just remember that your life is worth it and your advocate will probably be honored and more than willing to go the extra mile for you.

In addition, there are already—and in my view, there should be a dramatic increase in—professional patient advocates. Perhaps retired doctors would make great professional patient advocates. It would keep them in the health game and provide a credible counselor and liaison between the patient and the very busy, often very rigid, medical establishment. Some have worried that retired doctors might not make the best advocates, as they are likely to be the least enlightened about decision analysis, individualized treatment options, and the need for patient advocacy. But at the same time, they are intelligent and experienced people who may have some spare time on their hands. They might be willing to read pamphlets, take refresher courses, and take a primer in decision analysis—if only hospitals or other medical institutions would provide such things.

Once advocates become the norm rather than the exception, the really tough battle will be to eventually convince HMOs and insurance companies to pay for them—and that will likely take legislation. Enlightened legislators should be thinking about this and setting up hearings to weigh pros and cons. Needless to say, there will likely be an onslaught of contrary lobbying from HMOs, as they typically want to keep full control of and privacy for their hidden decision-making chambers and do not want to hear that patient interests should supersede their cost-cutting initiatives.

I came out of never-never land just as Sandra was explaining that I needed a CT scan[6] both to measure the extent of my disease and to use as a "before" picture against which we'd compare my progress once the treatments began. Terry and I asked about whether I should also go in for a PET scan,[7] which we had learned from the Web was an excellent and very sensitive supplementary diagnostic test. Sandra said, "Well, you may not be able to get the PET scan in time." "But isn't it important?" "Well, the results of PET scans are still controversial, but you're right: the more information we have, the better. However, you'll have to go to a private operator for it, because the hospital to which we normally refer patients for PET scans is backlogged, and you won't be able to get in there for weeks. I want to start your chemo next Tuesday, and we need all the results before then. It is urgent that we get this treatment started right away," she said. "We want to hit this cancer and hit it again and hit it again. We want to drive it down and knock it out." "Well, when will you get the bone marrow biopsy results back so that you know whether I have cancer in my bone marrow?" I asked. "You have cancer in your bone marrow," she confirmed. "Mantle cell lymphoma is typically everywhere almost all the time, even at the onset." I knew that I had met my match in this disease.

Prognosis: The News May Be Better Now

Sandra explained that the fact that I had lumps both above and below my diaphragm was a good indication that I had cancer in my marrow and that it was already a stage IV cancer. "Is that the worst prognosis?" I asked. "Well, all cancers can potentially go through four stages, with four being the worst, but for mantle cell, reaching stage IV is pretty common." Sandra wouldn't talk about the probability of survival. All she said was, "Don't read the Web; it'll depress you. What we do is too new to be found there, and it's vastly better."

The Internet is home to a huge amount of data on clinical trials and new treatments, but the information is not centralized or completely up-to-date—nor is most of it written in a way the average Joe can understand. In my own search for information, I spent countless hours (and Terry spent twice countless hours) online, jumping from cancer Web site to cancer Web site, sometimes to no avail. Most sites containing clinical trials databases were months behind in listing new clinical trials, and none included *all* the trials currently under way. Even the National Cancer Institute's Web site (http://www.cancer.gov) fails to list some private clinical trials sponsored by pharmaceutical and other companies. To compound the problem, some cancer Web sites give information that just isn't true or has never been tested. In a 2004 article in the *Annals of Oncology*,[8] it was reported that the most popular Web sites giving advice on "alternative" or "complementary" cancer treatments were actually a *risk* to cancer patients. The thirty-two Web sites studied listed cancer "cures" ranging from shark cartilage to mistletoe, none of which had been scientifically proven to work—by clinical trials *or* by Bayesian methods. Three of the sites went so far as to discourage patients from pursuing traditional cancer treatments, and one site advised against taking doctors' advice. Although I advocate getting involved in your treatments, it would be foolhardy, in my view, to ignore your doctor. Challenge, question, and cajole your doctor—but never snub her!

The good news is that the treatments for your cancer may be improved and your prognosis may be better than the Web would lead you to believe. Your doctor should know how to sort bogus data points from credible ones and could very well have information about clinical trials and improved treatments that are so new that they cannot yet be found on the Web. Your doctor may have learned of new treatments from trials that he or she or another doctor in the same hospital or medical facility was conducting, from outside trials, or from attending a medical conference where not-yet-published results were presented. The National Institutes of Health (NIH) has produced detailed requirements regarding the dissemination of clinical trials data, and one of them states that the institution sponsoring the study should distribute data on the study's findings to all relevant health care professionals, either prior to or concurrent with the public dissemination of the data. In many cases, your doctor will receive these data well before the majority of the public and well before they are published in medical journals. In fact, the *Journal of the American Medical Association*, a highly esteemed publication, states: "In situations where there is an immediate public health need for the information, there should be no delay in its release even if this release antedates AMA journal publication." Other journals have similar policies. In choosing a doctor, you will want one who seeks out such information, not one who is too busy to keep up with the literature or learn new techniques or who sticks to old-fashioned or familiar protocols.

It should also be encouraging to you as a patient that data from clinical trials are being incorporated into the practice of oncology more quickly than ever before, which can only improve your chances of remission. However, this is no reason to assume that diligence on your and your advocate's part is not necessary, because not all medical institutions have followed the trend of better and more rapid integration of new clinical trials data. As I learned from Harvey Fineberg, the head of the Institute of Medicine, some hospitals and clinics are not using clinical trials data at all, or at least not nearly as much as they should. In fact, some doctors are operating solely on the basis of their experiences with their last five patients. He gave a striking example: Suppose you're in rural Nebraska, where there are two cancer doctors treating every cancer case in four counties. It is possible that these doctors are out of touch with recent medical innovations and may not have read medical literature for years. Do you really want these doctors making up their own protocols? The process by which these docs may draw inferences could very well be ad hoc, unstructured, and highly error prone. Harvey said he does advocate the use of formal Bayesian procedures such as decision analysis and individualized treatment and testing, which offer a much more rigorous and transparent framework for making judgments about the likely consequences of a treatment choice for a particular patient. But at the same time, doctors need to begin from a solid foundation. For the hypothetical doctors in Nebraska, if Bayesian updating is not an option, proceeding via information provided by clinical trials sure beats winging it. I certainly agree with Harvey's logic.

In addition, even if your doctor is diligent, there is so much new cancer treatment information being released from day to day that it is possible—even likely—that your doctor just hasn't gotten word of a specific study or simply can't keep track of all the newly published results. Therefore, if you come across something interesting in your Web or other searching, gather as much information on it as you can and bring it to your next appointment. Your findings might just result in a new or at least an improved protocol for you and your fellow patients. It did for me.

Just remember, even when you come across legitimate new data on trials and treatments, a statistic is only a statistic. If you are confronted with daunting numbers on median mortality, remember that they are for the average patient, which you may not necessarily be. Stephen Jay Gould's essay "The Median Isn't the Message," which I mentioned in the preface, provides enlightening words on this subject. When Gould began reading about the "median mortality of eight months" for his cancer, he wrote:

My first intellectual reaction was: fine, half the people will live longer; now what are my chances of being in that half. I read for a furious and nervous hour and concluded, with relief: damned good. I possessed every one of the characteristics conferring a probability of longer life: I was young; my disease had been recognized in a relatively early stage; I would receive the nation's best medical treatment; I had the world to live for; I knew how to read the data properly and not despair.

Another technical point then added even more solace. I immediately recognized that the distribution of variation about the eight-month median would almost surely be what statisticians call "right skewed." (In a symmetrical distribution, the profile of variation to the left of the central tendency is a mirror image of variation to the right. In skewed distributions, variation to one side of the central tendency is more stretched out—left skewed if extended to the left, right skewed if stretched out to the right.) The distribution of variation had to be right skewed, I reasoned . . . there isn't much room for the distribution's lower (or left) half—it must be scrunched up between zero and eight months. But the upper (or right) half can extend out for years and years. . . .

The distribution was indeed, strongly right skewed, with a long tail (however small) that extended for several years above the eight month median. I saw no reason why I shouldn't be in that small tail. . . .

Gould's next, and perhaps most important point, also applies to median medical statistics: A statistical distribution only explains a specific circumstance or set of circumstances. In the case of most cancers, that distribution will describe success rates based on traditional treatments. But if any of the variables on which the distribution is based are changed (e.g., if a nonconventional treatment is used), the distribution could be very different—and perhaps much better.

Proof Positive

Sandra finished up with me and promised to have everything ready for my chemotherapy session the following Tuesday. I then went in for my CT scan, which was surprisingly easy. A nurse inserted an IV into my arm that pulsed a liquid contrast medium through my body, the scanner took ten minutes' worth of pictures, and I was done. I felt a slight hot flash when the IV liquid began running through my veins, but the procedure wasn't painful. I wasn't quite finished for the day, though. After the CT scan, I had another nuclear medicine test, a multiple gated acquisition (MUGA) scan to determine the "ejection fraction" of my heart—in short, how well my heart was pumping. It would be used as a benchmark for comparison after my treatment had started. As we had learned in our research, chemotherapy treatments can reduce a patient's heart ejection fraction, which can make life harder after treatment.

We found a private PET scan lab in San Jose and went there the next day. After I had been injected with a radioactive substance, the technician asked Terry to leave the room, since I was so "hot" (radioactive) that she shouldn't be exposed to me. The half-life of the stuff was only about twenty minutes, so it would be fine for Terry to be near me when the test was done. The PET scan was like a very slow CT scan. I lay on my back on a very slowly moving bench and was threaded through a donut-shaped set of receivers that were making a computer map of my radioactive emissions. Later on, the technician showed us the PET scan results, and they were nothing short of shocking. My lymph nodes, liver, spleen, bone marrow, and entire lymphatic system were all clearly highlighted in the three-dimensional outline of my body. I couldn't imagine there was a more convincing diagnostic out there. Although I didn't think the tech was supposed to show us the results—after all, according to medical dogma, only doctors were supposed to reveal such information to patients—it eliminated any remaining denial I had about my cancer and actually served as a motivator for me to fight and fight hard.

My insurance company balked at paying for the PET scan, but after some fighting on the phone with various agents, it paid a few thousand dollars, and Terry and I covered the difference when the bill came a month later. If I'd been a struggling, low-wage worker not vested in medical insurance, it's very unlikely that I would have been able to afford the several thousand dollars we paid for that important test.

Although I normally try to take a long-term view of any situation, at that stage in my illness, I was living from test to test and focusing on getting through one day at a time.

5 | "Once Per Lethal Disease": Coping with Chemo

DESPITE HAVING LEARNED from the Web that chemo is unpleasant at best and having pored over Lance Armstrong's wrenching (and retching) stories of his struggle to maintain his strength and equilibrium as his body was being infiltrated by these poisons, my chemo started out very well. The nurses, who were more than willing to answer all my questions, patiently explained what they were doing and outlined what was going to happen throughout the chemo process. About the only question they deflected was: How likely is it that the treatments would work? That was indeed the million-dollar question.

"Some Patients React"

After getting my IV of Benadryl and feeling the chain mail suit of grogginess descend, as described in chapter 1, I prepared myself for initiation into the world of chemotherapy, waiting for the first bottle of chemicals to enter my veins. I had seen other patients getting infused while settled in vinyl-upholstered "easy chairs" with two wide arms that patients could rest theirs on while connected to a maze of tubes and pumps, and I assumed that my treatment would be the same. But once I saw my chemo chemicals, I realized that there was a huge difference. Most of the chemicals the other patients were getting came in collapsible plastic bags, sometimes accompanied by a one-liter bag of saline solution that would also be injected to keep the patient hydrated. What I first got was a chemical that came in what looked like a glass seltzer bottle that tapered to a point where one end of a tube could be plugged into it. The other end of the tube would be attached to me so that the medicine could be dripped into my system. But my bottle was so big—it held 750 milliliters, about the amount of fluid in an ordinary wine bottle—relative to the others I'd seen that it became quite clear to me that I was going to be there a long time. Very long.

The nurses started the drip, and the magical potion flowed into me at a rate of 50 milliliters per hour, which, if divided into 750, would imply that I was going to be there for 15 hours waiting for this upside-down wine bottle to empty. I was supposed to get not just that first chemical that day, but three more as well! The infusion center was open only until 8:00 p.m., and it was already 2:00 p.m.; I just couldn't get the arithmetic to work. I tried to overcome my Benadryl fog and asked the nurse about it. She replied, "Don't worry; we'll increase the flow rate once we're sure that your body can tolerate the medicine, and eventually, we'll reach a flow rate of a few hundred milliliters per hour and get it finished in two or three hours. We should even have time for the rest of the meds afterward; they usually go much quicker." "Why do you have to start out so slowly?" I asked. I got a slightly evasive answer in return: "Some patients react; it's just better that way." "React?" I asked. "Just let us know if you feel chills, queasiness, or anything else unusual, and we'll be right over." I gave a halfhearted smile and focused on the slowly emptying bottle.

The chemical seeping into my veins was Rituxan, the drug that our research had told us was critical to the success of the Stanford protocol on non-Hodgkin's B-cell lymphoma. I remembered Michael Jacobs saying, "At least it isn't a T-cell cancer," when he first called to give me my diagnosis, and I learned that part of the reason he said that was because of this chemical, recently developed by IDEC Pharmaceuticals, a biotech company founded by Ron Levy and Richard Miller, Sandra Horning's husband and a postdoctoral Fellow in Levy's lab in the early 1980s. (The other reason Michael was happy I didn't have a T-cell cancer was because T-cell lymphomas tend to have worse prognoses. [Fortunately, T-cell cancers are rarer than B-cell cancers.] B-cell lymphomas, with the exception of mantle cell lymphoma, my disease, tend to be more amenable to treatments. But even mantle cell lymphoma is more sensitive to a variety of different chemotherapy treatments than many T-cell cancers.) Using knowledge of cellular and molecular biology, Levy, along with IDEC, invented an approach that literally trained a patient's body to turn its own immune fighting capacity against the cancer-contaminated B cells. Since B cells are actually infection fighters themselves, when they harbor cancer, the immune system may not treat them as the enemy. (There is a great debate about that, discussed later.) So the invasion-killer defenses that the immune system deploys to deal with bacteria and other foreign proteins that make us sick are not usually as effective against our own B cells, even if they're cancerous. That's probably a good thing, because if we routinely fought off our own B cells, we would be depriving our blood of some of its infection fighters.

So how did scientists find a way to make a cancer patient's immune system more effectively attack its own cancerous B cells, the stealth bombers of non-Hodgkin's patients' immune systems that can fly below the radars of their immune defenses? The trick was to find a protein, known as a monoclonal antibody,[1] that fit perfectly onto a B cell receptor known as a CD-20 site. The antibody attaches to the B cell much as a NASA spaceship would dock at a space station; it requires a perfect fit of ship and station for a leakproof match. The idea is that once the antibody is glued to the B cells, the immune system will recognize them as invaders and go after them.

Rituximab, the monoclonal antibody that evolved out of this research, was being marketed under the name Rituxan by IDEC together with Genentech, now a leading Bay Area biotechnology company. A treatment-sized dose of Rituxan for a patient like me consisted of 750 milliliters of clear-looking liquid loaded with billions of these proteins, each of which had "docking ends" that would attach chemically to the CD-20 receptors of my B cells.

Since my cancer cells were B cells plagued with out-of-control growth that could eventually crowd out all the other cells in my marrow that I needed to keep my immunities up, it was essential to kill those cancer cells. Unfortunately, the monoclonal antibody would attach to the CD-20 receptors on *all* my mature B cells, the good ones and the bad ones, so while my immune system was going to knock out cancer, it would knock out the healthy B cells as well. Fortunately, only mature B cells have CD-20 receptors, so even after the Rituxan, I'd be left with some immature B cells that could grow up and eventually replenish the supply—hopefully none being cancerous. But still, Rituxan was a high-tech biochemical miracle. Without causing damage to my heart, lungs, or nerves, as other toxins in my chemo cocktail would, this immunotherapy would attack the cancer throughout my marrow and lymph nodes.[2]

After all we had read about the benefits of Rituxan, Terry and I were surprised to learn that there are no long-term data indicating that giving mantle cell lymphoma patients Rituxan in addition to a traditional chemotherapy treatment is any better than the traditional treatment alone. However, there are no frequency data indicating the reverse (that traditional chemo is better than chemo plus Rituxan); in fact, with the exception of my current learning experience (see chapter 19) and a few small studies (one of which is discussed in chapter 17), there are almost no data at all. However, I'd be willing to bet—in fact, have bet my life on it—that as frequency data become available, Rituxan will be shown to be helpful both in combination with traditional chemotherapy and especially as a maintenance therapy after chemotherapy.

After an hour of feeling fuzzy and a little bored and wondering whether I was really going to be waiting for my wine bottle to drain for the next fifteen hours or if I was going to be sent home and asked to come back the next day, a nurse came in and upped the drip to 75 milliliters per hour. *Well, that's better*, I thought to my hazy-brained self sarcastically. *Now I can get out in a mere ten hours*. After another thirty or forty minutes, the nurse returned and said, "Hey, you're doing fine. Let's go to 100." "Why not double the 75 to 150?" I asked, feeling confident. "Your body is more likely to accept Rituxan the first time you're exposed to it if the drip rate is increased very gradually. Trust me, we know from experience." I agreed that 100 would be a good choice. Before leaving the room, the nurse again warned me to watch out for chills and nausea—"you know, flulike symptoms."

With all the liquid I was getting, frequent bathroom breaks were necessary, but my Benadryl chain mail made me uncomfortable navigating alone down the long hall that led to the restroom, especially since the IV had to come with me. I didn't mention it, but I guess I must have looked concerned, because as soon as I started to stand up, Terry grabbed my right arm, saying, "Let's just do this together." The thought that I would fall down and rip the IV out of my arm was more than incentive enough for me to overcome any foolish macho notions that might have prevented me from asking for assistance just to walk to the bathroom. Fortunately, I didn't need any help once there, just back and forth.

As we walked back from the bathroom, I began to feel just a little bit queasy. "It's getting difficult to walk," I said to Terry, confessing that I was feeling light-headed and felt a spell of nausea coming on, thanks to all the drugs and my changing positions. "Just take it easy," she said as I got back into the chair, "and don't keep any information to yourself. Tell us everything you're feeling."

Well, in the next two minutes, I couldn't have kept any information to myself if I had tried. My entire body started to shake, my teeth chattered, and my face turned white. Terry ran for the nurse and came back with her and a bucket just in time. The nurse cut the drip to zero.

For the next ten minutes, life was pure hell—just as Lance Armstrong's account suggested it would be. The nurses dripped something into my IV to calm me down, and it seemed to work. In another half hour, I started to feel a little bit more normal, though still very shaky in the pins. I looked warily up at the bottle of save-my-life fluid and realized that I had only gotten through about 150 milliliters. At a flow rate of zero, I'd be there until my funeral, but the hospital wouldn't be able to accommodate that, given that this particular wing was to close in three hours. "I need this stuff," I told the nurse. "Can we turn it back on?" "Yes, let's turn it back on slowly. And don't worry, Steve. From what I've seen, it's only the first day, and especially the first few hours, that are the most difficult. You'll get through this," she reassured me.

"You'll Get Through This"

The nurse started the drip again at 25 milliliters per hour, and I thought, *Great, I'll be in the hospital for two days*. But then, after twenty minutes, she came back and upped it to 50, and after another half hour, back to 75. Then, she came back with the intention of increasing the drip to 100 milliliters per hour, and I got cold feet. "100 is what took me out the first time," I said, "so maybe we should go to 90 or 95?" "Good idea," she said. So, I screwed up my courage, looked at my watch, and, chain mail and all, calculated that I'd need another seven hours to empty the bottle. I was bound and determined to get every drop of the liquid and the billions of proteins it contained into my body, because I knew that I had a lot of B cells that needed to come in contact with the proteins and then get attacked by my own immune system if I was to survive the disease.

The next three hours seemed to drag on forever, but it appeared that my body was accepting the Rituxan. I never felt great, but there was no more violent retching, shaking, or nausea, just that ever-present underlying queasiness. I didn't want to get up and go to the bathroom despite the gobs of fluid running into my system, for I was afraid that would trigger another episode, so I sat there grinning and bearing it as my bladder got fuller and fuller.

Finally, around 8:00 p.m., the nurse said, "We have to go home. This section has to close." "You mean I can't even get the whole bottle today?" I asked. "Oh, we're going to get all of this into you," she said. "We have a 23-hour section of the hospital, and you can go over there." "Twenty-three hour?" Terry asked. "Yeah, it's for patients who haven't actually been admitted. They can stay for up to 23 hours—some bureaucratic thing that allows us to handle people in your situation without having to go and register them and deal with all kinds of hassles." It sounded pretty reasonable to us.

"Okay, I'm ready to go," I said. "Okay," said the nurse. "Stand up. We'll support you while you walk." "Are you sure I can do this?" I asked. "Of course I am," she said. "You just got through three hours of chemo without any more episodes; the walk won't matter." I decided to trust her, and there was some urgency in doing so, as my bladder was about to burst. We headed to the 23-hour section, making a pit stop at the bathroom on the way, and I reached my new room no queasier than when I started the journey. I began to believe that, sooner or later, I might actually get through the first day. I tried not to think about the fact that I'd have to repeat this procedure every three weeks.

As the night wore on, nurses from different shifts came in to check on Terry and me. I watched the large bottle of Rituxan drain, going from two-thirds full to half full to one-third full. Sometime around 11:00 p.m., the fluid actually reached the conical section of the upside-down bottle, and I could see the light at the end of the tunnel (and through the bottle!). A nurse came in and said, "You'll be able to go home soon," and I replied, "Not until I get every drop of this stuff." She said she was going to be there all night anyway, and it didn't matter if we stayed the whole time. Finally, a little after midnight, the drip stopped, and the whole wine bottle's worth of clear, life-saving proteins were circulating in my body. I was exhausted.

"Do I get my other chemos now?" I asked. "No," the nurse said. "We need someone who has been specially trained in vesicants to administer them, and all those people have gone home now. You'll have to come back tomorrow to get those." "Vesicants?" "Yes, the other chemo chemicals you're going to get, at least some of them, are so toxic that if even one drop spills on your skin or the nurse's, it will burn a hole in it just like an acid would, so it's better to have it infused by somebody with special training." That certainly didn't make me look forward to coming back the next day: If one drop was so caustic on the outside of the body, I could only imagine what it was going to do to my insides.

We got a call from the hospital the next morning, and I went in, accompanied by Terry, at 1:00 p.m. to get the remainder of the CHOP protocol—the first-generation chemo treatment I was being given in addition to the Rituxan, which consisted of four different drugs: cyclophosphamide (or Cytoxan), hydroxy-daunorubicin (also called doxorubicin or Adriamycin), Oncovin (also called vincristine), and prednisone. First I was given my IV feeding of Benadryl; then Kytril, an antinausea medicine;[3] then some other things I don't even remember; and then the chain mail descended. As I was entering my haze phase, a nurse came in carrying two horse-sized syringes filled with a bright orange-red liquid that looked like syrupy Kool-Aid. "What's that stuff?" I groggily blurted out. "It's Adriamycin, a very common chemotherapy drug for lymphoma and leukemia." "Is that a vesicant?" I asked. "Why, yes," she responded, somewhat surprised that I knew what it was and what it meant and that I could remember it while under the influence. "I've been watching my IV fittings carefully," I reported, "to make sure that the tubes don't leak—I gather this stuff is no good for either of us if it gets loose." "Indeed, you're right," she said, "but it won't. Don't worry. It never has in all the years I've been doing this."

She disconnected the Benadryl tube and connected me to another tube that was attached to the syringe filled with the iridescent red-orange vesicant. Adriamycin is so viscous—and toxic, too, I suppose—that it can't be dripped like some other drugs can. Instead, it is injected. The nurse put one hand on the tube, the other on a plunger, and very, very slowly injected the vile-looking stuff into my IV. When the first tube was finished, the fittings were carefully disconnected, cleaned, and reconnected. The second syringe was connected, and the process was repeated. I worried that if the nurse pushed too hard on the plunger and the fluid was viscous enough, it might create enough back pressure to pop the fittings and send Adriamycin flying all over the place, but I figured it would be insulting to mention it. I couldn't imagine that anyone trained in vesicants and aware of the risks faced by both the patient and the specialist administering them wouldn't be aware of that possibility. This probably explained why the nurse injected the orange goo so slowly; it took twenty minutes to inject both tubes of it into my body even though each contained no more than 50 milliliters of fluid.

When the nurse had finished administering the Adriamycin, she brought out a very small syringe that contained a little bit of clear fluid. I was already smiling, thinking this would be quick and easy, but then I learned that the vincristine I was about to get was also a vesicant, so once again I scrutinized every part of the process.

"Isn't vincristine one of the oldest chemos out there? It comes from a plant, the Madagascar periwinkle, right?" Terry asked. "Why, yes," the nurse said, sounding surprised. "It's been around a long time, it's very effective, and it *did* come from some tropical flower." I then remembered some of Tom Lovejoy's speeches I had heard about the need to preserve primary forests, particularly in tropical areas. There are millions of species in the world that we know about, and many millions more not yet discovered, and Tom likes to point out that if we wipe them out before we even have the chance to learn about them, we could destroy the next cure for cancer without even knowing it. Ironically, these plants, which have the potential to improve societies' standards of living, are being destroyed by the increasing number of people demanding higher standards of living without giving adequate foresight to protecting nature. The environmentalist in me was quite pleased to know that the chemical I was getting, which was so instrumental in reversing the scourge of childhood leukemia and other diseases, like my own, came from a flower that was threatened but saved just in time, when its incredible value to the human race was discovered.

Informed Consent

Even after all my sleuthing, I was not aware of the potential neurological side effects of vincristine until after the fact. The biggest danger is that vincristine can trigger peripheral neuropathy, a disorder that causes tingling, numbness, and sometimes pain in the extremities. Vincristine was part of the standard protocol at Stanford and elsewhere, and I'm sure that when I signed all the paperwork before undergoing chemotherapy, there was probably some fine print containing such information that I failed to read. I was nervous about signing the paperwork for this very reason, but I figured the forms were like those signed by people about to have surgery, indemnifying the institutions by conceding the patient is aware of the risks of the procedure.

When I found out about the possible side effects, I realized once again how important it is for patients to ask questions and stay as well informed as possible about their diseases and the pros and cons of various treatments. I decided—though in retrospect in this instance—that the benefits of vincristine outweighed the costs in my particular case, as I knew we needed to kill my cancer cells. Clearly, the experience the doctors had had with the multiple chemo agents in the CHOP protocol combined with Rituxan suggested that it would give me the highest chance of success, even if there was then very little frequency data to prove it. However, I realized that the benefits might not always outweigh the costs in future treatment situations, and from then on, I tried to remember to ask Sandra about the side effects of different procedures and drugs at each turn so that I could be an effective member of our decision-making team. I suggest that all patients or their advocates do the same.

—⊣ ⊢—

The chemo session ended with a 50-milliliter plastic drip bag of an innocent-looking nonvesicant called Cytoxan. I had a hard time believing that it was any less poisonous than the gooey blood-orange vesicants I'd just been given, considering that its last name was only one letter off from "toxin." The drug's primary job was to kill cells in the marrow, formally termed "myeloablative action," and since (though I did not yet have exact figures) 40 percent of my bone marrow cells were plagued with mantle cell lymphoma, scouring my marrow was essential to saving my life. Like vincristine, Cytoxan had its dangers; it was known to deteriorate heart and lung condition, so once again, the cost-benefit calculus was not going to see me getting away scot-free.

Amazingly, all three chemo chemicals were infused in less than two hours, and I suffered no side effects other than the grogginess from the Benadryl, which still hadn't quite worn off as we walked out that afternoon. What a contrast to the Rituxan nightmare the day before! "We'll see you in three weeks," said the nurse. "And don't worry—very few people have the same reaction to the Rituxan the second time around." She unplugged my IVs, gave me some informational brochures, and told me that I was to take the prednisone, the "P" in the CHOP protocol, in pill form at home for the next five days. This powerful steroid would help my body cope with the chemo agents as my liver detoxified them.

When Misery Is a Good Sign

As we were walking through the hospital door toward the parking lot, who should be walking in but Sandra Horning. "Hi, Sandra," I said. "We *finally* finished with the CHOP a few minutes ago." "I heard you had a pretty hard time with the Rituxan yesterday," she said, surprising me with her cheerful tone. I nodded. "Actually, it's a good sign when you get sick like that." "How so?" I asked incredulously. "Well, it means that your immune system was activated all at once, just like it would be if you were getting the flu, and it immediately began attacking your B cells because it thought they were invaders once the monoclonal antibodies attached to them. The side effects you experienced suggest that the drug is working. So it's actually a good thing that you reacted the way you did. It's also a good indication that the Rituxan will do its job throughout your treatment." "I wish I had known that in advance!" I said. "Well, not everybody has such a strong reaction to the drugs, and we don't like to scare anybody too badly beforehand. Just be glad that it suggests your chemo is working," she reiterated.

What Do You Really Want to Know in Advance?

Is there a balance between knowing what is most important and not knowing so much as to invoke the power of suggestion (i.e., the "reverse placebo effect")? I cannot answer this question for everyone and believe it varies on a case-by-case basis. Each patient and his or her advocate will have to grapple with this issue and make the decision that is right for them based on the patient's preferences. When it came to my own choice between blissful ignorance and informed worry, I guess I preferred to err on the side of more knowledge. I figured that being well informed could help me face a problem better and make the right choices. Personally, I'd have welcomed the terrible side effects had I known they indicated that my treatment was working. It is easier for many of us to accept hardship when we understand the benefits, so for me, the reverse placebo effect gets trumped by the "know-what's-happening" effect. But what works for me might not work for everyone. These knowing versus not knowing situations are ripe for intervention by an advocate.

Despite thinking I wanted all the information possible about my disease and my particular case, there were certain facts that I *didn't* know, and it was probably for the best. Neither Terry nor I was ever told at the outset just how much of my bone marrow cells (40 percent) were infected by lymphoma, and I'm not sure I would have wanted to know. Knowing it wouldn't have changed the treatment plan, so perhaps the docs were right to "forget" to tell us when the results of the bone marrow biopsy came in. However, other details about my diagnosis and treatments that the docs chose to omit might have changed Terry's and my decisions. There was no telling whether the docs—the only ones in possession of certain information—made the same decisions Terry and I would have made had we been given those facts. I don't know whether our value systems and use of decision analysis would have led to different decisions about my treatment regimen or not, but given that this risk exists, I prefer full disclosure and would again put worries about any "reverse placebo effect" in second place.

Another approach, as I suggested earlier, would be for the doctors to tell difficult information to an advocate, who could then, knowing the patient's general value system and orientation, decide how much to tell the patient, while at the same time working with the doctors for treatment planning purposes and sparing the patient that stress. This in fact happens in many medical situations today. Often, the physician will share information about a patient's diagnosis and prognosis with family members and not directly with the patient, the idea being that the family members will best know how to relay the news to the patient. Perhaps that is the best way for some patients to navigate this treacherous trade-off between full disclosure and becoming overburdened with worrisome facts.

Whose Decision Is It Anyway?

All these deliberations brought back a memory from many years ago when I first confronted this "to know or not to know" trade-off. My spouse at that time was pregnant with our daughter, and we contemplated amniocentesis.[4] The doctors advised against it, as she was thirty-three years old, and thirty-five was the minimum age at which they recommended amnio. I foolishly left it unquestioned. Two years later, when my ex-wife was thirty-five and pregnant with our son, the doctor said amnio was a "borderline decision." So I finally asked, "What is it about thirty-five years old that is a threshold for a go/no-go decision for amnio?" "Oh that's simple," he said. "At thirty-five the curves cross." "What curves?" I asked with wrinkled brow. "The risk of spontaneous abortion of the fetus becomes equal—on average, of course—to the risk of serious genetic defects (like Down's syndrome) in the fetus." I was shocked and angry. "You mean to tell me you are making this fundamental value choice for the patients without even telling us the trade-offs? Suppose we were religious people opposed to all forms of abortion—then there would be no age at which we'd risk spontaneous abortion as a side effect. On the other hand, suppose we thought it was immoral to bring a horribly disadvantaged child into the world, and we didn't oppose abortions. That decision should be the parents' choice because these trade-offs are personal value judgments, not medical science. All medicine can do is tell us the numbers—probabilities for abortion, genetic defects, etc.—but to make the choice is the patients' right." I was steamed. How could these professionals make the value judgments on difficult moral issues for the parents?

—| |—

Sandra accompanied us outside, reminding me to be certain to take the prednisone and the antinausea medicine. "Stay with the regimen," she said. "The Compazine really helps, but if you wait too long between doses, you'll feel queasy all over again, and once that starts, it's hard to reverse. Just stay vigilant." I promised I would.

"One more thing, Sandra," I blurted out as she was heading into the hospital. "My friends want to take me out to dinner in a couple days. Is it safe to go?" "It's really up to you. It all depends on how you feel," she said. "Don't push it, but if you feel okay, go ahead. Just take it easy, and don't drink too much." "You mean I can't have wine?" I asked. "Not much." "Then I'm not sure it's worth going out!" I quipped. "Well, if it's really great stuff, measure out two fingers' worth in your glass—just enough to get a taste," she said, holding her middle and index fingers together horizontally. "But remember, your liver is already working overtime to detoxify some pretty potent chemicals, so you don't want to over-complicate its job with too much alcohol." I thanked her, and in reality, I actually appreciated that she had explained her reasoning for limiting my alcohol intake; as a result, I'd be more willing to avoid the wine, even though I knew it would be wonderful, be-cause every time Terry and I go out to dinner with our friends Paul and Anne Ehrlich, we try fun wines.

I went home, clueless as to how I was going to endure multiple rounds of chemo. Exhaustion, nausea, neutropenia,[5] severe allergic reaction, acid reflux, and altered appetite and tastes were among the lovely side effects detailed in the documents the hospital had given us and in what we had read on the Web. One bout of such symptoms would be bearable, but two or three or five or more? I grimaced at the thought.

I stayed home for a day, just in case something went wrong, and Terry stayed with me, working from her home office. Surprisingly, every time I got up and went to the phone or even checked my e-mail, I felt pretty normal. I was still plagued by an underlying queasiness, which I could suppress by taking the Compazine and some other drugs, but amazingly enough, I really didn't feel too weird. I figured that part of the reason I felt okay was that I was taking 100 milligrams of prednisone per day for five straight days, and it seemed to be preventing delayed allergic reactions to the chemo agents and lessening the side effects of the other drugs I was taking. The problem was that 100 milligrams was a very large dose, and the prednisone itself was known to cause side effects, including a massive increase in appetite and a change in mood—mostly in the direction of hyperactivity, the last thing I or anybody around me needed!

The nurses had explained that after about four or five days, my liver would have detoxified most of the chemo chemicals, and then I'd be able to stop taking the prednisone. "Don't you have to taper off prednisone?" Terry had asked the doctors earlier. "Well, if you take it for a long time, you do," they said, "but after only five days on it, we just tell patients to stop, and most people tolerate it." So, I was going to drop from 100 milligrams of prednisone per day to zero, which, according to Terry's Web research and my medical encyclopedia, was an absolute no-no, as prednisone is a slow-taper drug regardless of the length of time it's taken. Going "cold turkey" could cause serious psychological side effects, like depression, as well as physical discomforts.

I called Gary Wynbrandt, a psychiatrist in Menlo Park, and I asked him about the 100-to-zero prednisone non-taper that I would experience in a few days. He laughed. "I don't think anybody should be around you in the days after that happens." "What symptoms should I expect?" I asked. "You can probably blame any uncharacteristically strong reactions to events or situations on the withdrawal. You'll get through it, like the docs said, but with such a significant drop-off, there's no way you'll be free of side effects in the two or three days afterward, so be careful, and try to recognize situations in which you could potentially overreact to stimulation." I also checked in with Sharon Conarton, a former nurse and psychotherapist in Denver, whom I knew while living there. Her answer mirrored Gary's: "Not sure too many people should be around you the day after you go cold turkey!"

The Importance of Feeling Human

On the second day after chemo, I felt fairly good, although I always felt a little nauseated in the morning after the Compazine had worn off. (I was learning to get up in the middle of the night to take one.) Terry and I decided to stick with our plan to go out to dinner with Paul and Anne. They were concerned that I might be overdoing it, but I told them I was medically cleared for a few days until my white counts dropped too low the second week (recall the parabola of chapter 1), so as long as I kept my wine consumption to a few centimeters in the bottom of my glass it was OK. They agreed to monitor my consumption, and we met up at one of our favorite restaurants. Paul was kind and ordered a mediocre wine so I wouldn't feel too bad, but I did cheat a little bit and drank three fingers worth rather than two over the course of the evening.

When the meal arrived and we all dug in, I immediately noticed that my sense of taste had gone haywire. The chemo had left me with a metallic taste in my mouth and made potatoes taste like cardboard, but, remarkably, it had little effect on my acid- and fruit-tasting capacity, so the wine still tasted like wine. *What a lucky break*, I thought to myself. I'd trade off lost enjoyment of potatoes to retained taste of wine in a microsecond!

When I mentioned my altered sense of taste, Terry said, "Yeah, they emphasized that over and over again on the Web, but I didn't want to tell you because if I did, I knew you'd be looking for it."

Now, even my own wife and advocate had joined the conspiracy of deciding what I needed to hear! But she was right. Had I been told, I probably would have been wary with every bite I took, which would have made eating much less fun from the get-go—and I needed all the fun I could get those days.

Finally, at the end of our very pleasant meal, the first occasion in weeks in which I felt like a human being out in the real world, and not a victim, I pulled my credit card out of my wallet. Our usual procedure was to split the bill 50–50 between my and Paul's credit cards. But there was no bill. Paul started to get up, and I looked at him, confused. "Paul, we haven't paid yet." "You're right. *We* haven't paid yet. The bill is taken care of." Then it dawned on me: "Why did you pay? We always split these!" I protested. "Don't worry about it," he said, helping Anne up. "C'mon, my credit card still works!" I bellowed. "Don't get too used to this," Paul said, smiling. "I only treat once per lethal disease."

We all cracked up over his usual intemperate wise-assed humor. What could I say? In fact, a few days later, when I lost nearly all my hair in the span of two days, and after that, when I was suffering through more nasty chemo moments, I would remember his feisty quip and immediately feel better. As the Web said, and as I was beginning to realize, a support group, formal or not, is absolutely essential to anyone facing a life-threatening medical situation and undergoing such harsh treatments. Terry was support group member number one, but my extended group helped not only me but her too, as the prime caretaker needs support as much as the patient. In fact, David Spiegel, a psychiatrist at Stanford University Medical Center with whom we met several times after my treatments, has shown in his research that cancer patients with support did better statistically than a group that didn't have much bolstering. If you are undergoing treatment, don't think it is an imposition to ask for human interaction—it might help save your life.

6 "How Can You Know I'm in Remission?"

DESPITE MY ROCKY START with chemotherapy, the rest of my chemo treatments were really pretty tolerable. I still went to work, ate like a horse (at least in the first week, while I was still taking the prednisone), and the only time I ever had to stay at home was during those few days after my first chemo session, when the results of my third blood test showed that I had a dangerously low white count—something that never happened again thanks to the Neupogen shots I had "earned."[1]

The Neupogen was delivered to my house by express courier in a temperature-controlled container and had to be put in the refrigerator immediately. There were explicit instructions on how to self-inject the Neupogen and how to have somebody else perform the injection. Not surprisingly, I recruited Terry to be my injector. The instructions recommended that the Neupogen be injected into the abdomen or thigh, but I didn't really want that. Years earlier, when Terry had phlebitis and I had to give her subdermal injections of anticoagulants, she wanted the shots in her abdomen, and just the thought of it made me squeamish. Still, I dutifully performed the stabbing ritual, feeling really bad if it drew blood or even a wince. Now it was her turn.

Terry was not looking forward to the jab job she inherited, but she had paid very careful attention to the nurses' instructions for administering the shots and agreed to do whatever would improve my chances. "I guess it's like giving the dog its shots, so I can manage," she rationalized. "Ah, so now my status is on par with the wolves," I mused. Earlier, we had to give one of our dogs subdermal injections for severe allergies, so we knew the drill: pinch a flap of skin, rub it with alcohol, put the needle in at a low angle, back it up to be sure you're not on a blood vessel, then slowly inject, pull out, apply alcohol again, and say you're sorry.

We agreed that the shots would go into the back of my arm because Terry would be able to get a good angle there and I wouldn't have to watch. Actually, our little ritual wasn't so bad, especially since I needed only a total of five shots after each chemo treatment. That proved to be enough to stimulate my stem cells to produce white blood cells for the two and a half weeks until my next chemo cycle, and I never again had the dramatically low white blood cell counts that I had after the first round.

While I was aware that the Neupogen was literally a lifesaver, it, too, was said to have costs: In addition to being an expensive, hard-to-get drug, the package insert that came with it warned that bone pain was not a rare side effect, although I never noticed it during my five-shot series. In fact, at the beginning of treatments, I seemed not to experience most of the many symptoms I was warned about, but my good fortune wasn't to last throughout my treatment.

A Wild Ride

Five days after my first chemo infusion, my 100-milligram daily dose of prednisone went to zero, as required by the Stanford protocol. Despite the warnings from Gary Wynbrandt and Sharon Conarton about weird mood or behavioral changes, I didn't notice any. At least not at first.

Two days after I stopped taking the prednisone, Terry and I were driving home. We live on a rather curvy street with blind driveways jutting off of it. Just a mile away, there is a four-lane highway with a 65-mile-an-hour speed limit. We often comment, sarcastically, that drivers confuse our street with the highway, as many pay no attention to the 35-mile-an-hour signs that line our twisty residential zone, and they pose a threat to the neighborhood. As we were cruising along (at the speed limit, of course) that particular day, a car raced up behind us and was virtually hugging our tail. Our narrow street has blind hills and double yellow lines— meaning no passing—but this jerk had the nerve to pass us on a hill, racing along, pedal to the metal, wanting to go 65 miles per hour, and two days into my prednisone withdrawal, no less!

I lost it. I said, "Get the license plate number. I'm going to find out where he lives and throw rocks through every window in his goddamn car. He should be machine-gunned!" Terry looked at me with wide eyes. "Wow." A few seconds passed in silence, and then I started to laugh, thinking of Gary's warning about strange behavior. Normally, I'd be angered by that kind of moronic stunt by a driver, but throwing rocks through his windows and machine-gunning him!?! That definitely went above and beyond any normal reaction to such an event. In fact, I could feel a strange mood brewing inside of me, and I felt as though I'd had another out-of-body experience. In my head, I was sitting in the back seat, looking at this lunatic in the passenger seat ranting and raving about one dangerous driver and considering biblical stoning—or its modern equivalent, courtesy of the gun lobby—to be an appropriate punishment.

"Whoa," I said. "I guess the therapists were right." Terry laughed but warned me to remain vigilant for the next day and a half, at which point the withdrawal effect was supposed to end. "Maybe you should stay home and avoid anybody who might annoy you," she said with a smile.

"Does That Mean I'm Cured?
Or Do I Need Maintenance Therapy?"

By the end of the first week after chemo, the harsh chemicals (other than Rituxan, which stays in one's system for months) were detoxified by my liver, which meant I could go off the Compazine and most of the other drugs designed to reduce the side effects of chemo. I actually felt pretty good. In fact, I began to wonder why people had so overstated the negative side effects of chemo; I was having a relatively easy go of it aside from some nausea from time to time and my entertaining overreactions to trivial stress for a day or two after I stopped taking the prednisone. Paul, Anne, Terry, and I still climbed up the Stanford Dish trail, which was part of a one-square-mile park located right behind our house. We'd walk several hundred feet up a hill with a big radio telescope dish on the top of it, and on a clear day, we'd get a beautiful view of the San Francisco Bay and the Santa Cruz Mountains. It was pretty steep to start, and I didn't feel up to doing it much the first week after chemotherapy, but once the detoxification was complete, I would go, and while not exactly sprinting, was able to make it. The more things I could do that were normal, the better I felt.

Of course, there was the ever-present concern about what was going to come next, how quickly my cancer was being brought under control, and, most important, if I would ever completely get rid of it. The more we read about mantle cell lymphoma, the less likely it seemed that a total cure was in the cards. It was well established in the medical literature that mantle cell lymphoma's indolent component was difficult to kill off entirely.

The more I learned about the Stanford protocol that was being used on me, the more I thought about the need for "maintenance therapy." Basically, the protocol called for four to six CHOPs (plus Rituxan), then a bone marrow transplant (actually, a "stem cell rescue"—more on that technicality later), followed by, I was told by my medical team, "nothing." "Does that mean I'm cured after the bone marrow transplant?" I wanted to know. "We never use the word 'cured'," Sandra said, "just remission. We're very hopeful you will have a long and strong remission." "But if a remission ends," I said, "that means that not all the cancer cells were killed by the chemos, the Rituxan, and the bone marrow transplant. There's a possibility that something could still get through." "That's true," Sandra said, "which is why we often use radiation in addition to high-dose chemotherapies and the bone marrow transplant. Lymphoma cells can hide in all sorts of inconspicuous places, like behind your eyeballs. The danger is that the blood-brain barrier can reduce the effectiveness of chemicals like Rituxan, and any cancer cells in your head may not be killed, but radiation helps to take care of them."

It was early in my treatment, and I wasn't thinking about a bone marrow transplant, and in fact, I had somehow rationalized to myself that I was going to react so well to the other treatments that I wouldn't even need one. Instead, what I wanted was "maintenance therapy." Here was my reasoning: In its acute phase, my cancer was life threatening; there were tens of billions of cancer cells floating around in my body. If the chemo didn't kill the disease completely but merely knocked my cancer cell count down into the thousands, and if those cells then doubled every month or two, I'd be right back where I started in a few years! In fact, some of the data that Terry was finding on the Web (and wasn't telling me about at that time) suggested precisely that: Roughly 50 percent of patients on this protocol lost remission at least once in a four-year period. *So, why not take a different tack*, I thought to myself, *and just presume that we have not wiped out the cancer completely? Every few months, we could just administer Rituxan, and perhaps a low-dose chemo, to beat back the smallish number of cancer cells.*

During my second appointment with Sandra and the Fellow, I voiced my thoughts. "It doesn't matter if you never cure my cancer. All we have to do is keep the malignant cell count below a dangerous level, so why not use a low-dose intervention on a regular basis at the end of the process, when you'd normally just sit back and wait?" Sandra, who is a pensive, thoughtful type, didn't react, but the Fellow had a strong opinion. "We have no data whatsoever to suggest that low-dose interventions would have any benefit, and operating without data would be foolhardy." "You don't have any data suggesting it doesn't work because when it was tried it didn't work, or because nobody's tried it?" "The latter," Sandra said, still thinking carefully about what I'd said. "So why would you assume it doesn't work if you haven't run the data to find out? Remember the old line: absence of evidence isn't evidence of absence! I'll volunteer, because when we reach the end of the protocol, I don't want to live each day wondering if I'm carrying cells that could multiply back into a serious disease any day." I remembered Sandra saying that second remissions were harder to achieve than firsts. Furthermore, a full comeback of the disease would require additional high-dose chemotherapy, which could cause further heart and lung damage—not exactly a good omen for long-term health. So why not maintenance therapy?

It was very difficult to talk through this one with the Fellow, for in his view, if there were no clinical trials data showing that a particular treatment worked, it would be idiotic to try. He had no desire to pioneer such a risky experiment. Sandra was more open, agreeing that in the absence of clinical trials data, performing decision analysis and tracing my and her treatment thought process from beginning to end were good tools for dealing with my disease. I was glad that she was receptive but frustrated that we hadn't had the one-hour conversation that I asked for on day one to discuss these long-term alternatives. There was no doubt in my mind that maintenance therapy was preferable to the formula prescribed by the standard protocol: beat the hell out of the cancer and me and then hang around and wait until a CT scan picks up signs of cancer again, which it won't do until there are half a billion malignant cells and a palpable lump, at which point it would be too late to get away with a low-dose intervention like maintenance therapy.

After much prodding, Sandra somewhat reluctantly agreed to schedule a meeting to sit down with Terry and me so that we could perform a decision analysis, in which we would draw flow charts of various treatment alternatives, filling in the probabilities of success of each alternative based on the intuitions of Sandra and her team. We all agreed that it made the most sense to meet an hour before my next chemo appointment would begin.

Every Last Cancer Cell

I was still feeling good after my third cycle of chemo. I'd already gotten used to the slight queasiness that always seemed to plague me in the first week after treatment, the prednisone withdrawal, and the five days of Neupogen shots. The blood test on the fourteenth day after chemo no longer reported that my white blood cell count was dangerously low, thanks to the Neupogen. Since I no longer had dangerously low white cell counts the second week after chemo, I got into the routine of scheduling all my wining and dining outings for the second and third weeks of the cycle, when my liver had much less detoxifying to do and I could at least have half a glass of wine with dinner. And Paul did keep his word—I only got one free dinner.

In what little spare time I had, I read more about microbiology and chemotherapy in preparation for our meeting with Sandra. Despite having been a ten-year member of Stanford's biology department, two-thirds of which is made up of microbiologists, my knowledge of microbiology was pretty abysmal—the only downfall of hanging out with the ecologically oriented members of the department. I took an interest in the microbiologists' research and areas of expertise that I never had previously. I found out about how T cells, B cells, and killer cells worked, learned what the monoclonal antibody was doing, and discovered a special technique known as PCR, polymerase chain reaction, that I thought might be able to help me.

PCR is basically a highly sensitive molecular-based diagnostic test that is becoming increasingly popular in biology departments and in medicine. It mimics the way DNA would naturally copy itself but does so in a test tube. Key to the copying are a group of enzymes called polymerases that are trained—using two stretches of DNA known as "primers"—to "photocopy" preexisting DNA molecules.[2] By multiplying small but unique sections of DNA, scientists may be able to detect patterns or abnormalities in a person's genetic code. In fact, PCR is already being used in medicine to identify various diseases. In oncology the technique is still uncommon, but I imagine it will become widespread with time. As scientists discover what types of DNA abnormalities characterize different cancers, primers may be developed that will provide diagnostic information and detect even minimal levels of residual cancer cells, even when the patient is, by other measures, in remission.

The primary drawback of PCR is that the polymerases can be trained to split and remake only a single molecule at a time, so it takes quite a while for technicians to construct a primer for an individual piece of DNA, like the one making up my cancer-ridden lymph nodes. Regardless of the hassle, I was beginning to think that PCR might be worth a shot. Terry and I had learned that a CT scan is a very crude measure of remission and that a comeback of my cancer would show up on the scan only when my cancer cells had multiplied significantly—into the hundreds of millions, at least. Thus, saying that I was in "remission" because the CT scan revealed nothing struck me as a fool's paradise. I wanted to know whether I had even one single cancer cell in every cc of blood they took out of me. I knew that the hospital's lab could do a test on my blood using PCR, which would give us a much more accurate read on my cancer cell count. I added this request to my list of items to discuss with Sandra.

Continuing on our quest to gather as much information as possible for our meeting with Sandra, Terry and I again focused on the prospect of maintenance therapy. At the suggestion of colleagues and friends connected with Stanford, I sent Ron Levy, co-inventor of Rituxan, an e-mail and told him of my proposal to be given maintenance therapy using Rituxan. I noted the skepticism I had met with, at least from the Fellow, when I mentioned it at my last appointment. I asked Ron whether it would make sense to continuously hammer down the number of cancer cells with low doses of Rituxan once my treatment was "finished." I quizzed him on why I should even bother with a bone marrow transplant that promised to trigger nasty side effects, ranging from an increased probability of contracting leukemia or developing cataracts to dying from the procedure (although my procedure was not going to be as risky as some, since I would get my own cleansed cells back, not somebody else's[3]). I explained my dilemma and asked for Ron's expert advice.

Ron replied promptly in a lengthy e-mail. In essence, he said that maintenance therapy was a new concept and that doctors at Stanford and elsewhere had very little experience with it; nobody knew how or if Rituxan would work as maintenance therapy. On the other hand, he thought that it sounded like a pretty sensible idea, and he would support it if I was in a position that I needed it. However, he was adamant about the bone marrow transplant: "Do the bone marrow transplant; it will dramatically improve your odds. You can think about maintenance therapy later on if the bone marrow transplant isn't completely successful."

Ron's sage counsel mirrored my own thoughts for the most part, although I certainly would have liked an excuse to get out of the bone marrow transplant, given how taxing I was learning it would be. Terry had been very upbeat about every aspect of my treatment, but every time the bone marrow transplant topic surfaced, she was silent and her brow became furrowed, which I took to mean that she knew more than I did about what it was going to be like. She denied it, but after ten years, I knew her well enough to understand that she was a very good barometer of reality in such situations.

The Doctor Is Busy—But It's Your Life

When the third chemo cycle came around, Terry and I arrived at the hospital at 7:50 a.m., and we had to wait outside until the doors to Oncology Day Care opened ten minutes later. As the first patient, I got my blood test quickly and didn't have to wait in line. Then Terry and I were ushered into a small exam room. We were used to long waits, but our whole point of arriving an hour before my 9:00 a.m. appointment that day was to make sure we had time to sit down with Sandra, and hopefully the Fellow, too, to do our decision analysis. However, the entire oncology ward seemed nearly deserted. A few doctors scurried quickly by the open door of our examination room, filing into and out of a conference room. Most patients had not yet arrived, and neither had the doctors. At 9:00 a.m., nurses started ushering patients into rooms, but still, there were no doctors to be seen. Finally, several *hours* later, Sandra's Fellow came in nonchalantly and mentioned that I should get a CT scan after my third chemo treatment to measure my progress. "Fine," I said, "but you missed our meeting this morning. Don't you remember that we had an appointment to discuss decision analysis and long-term treatments?" "Very busy day, staff meeting, just the way it gets around here," he answered hurriedly.

Terry was furious. She almost lost it as the Fellow was leaving, but I grabbed her arm and shook my head no. She couldn't believe the oncologists blew off the appointment, and neither could I, but we figured that they probably never wanted to have it in the first place.

Sandra's failure to show up for our meeting felt like a major defeat to me as a patient and as a fellow professor and human being. Terry and I were angry, hurt, and discouraged, and our first inclination—after letting Sandra know exactly how we felt—was to give up on scheduling the appointment. However, we realized that giving up on meeting with Sandra to discuss the best course of treatment for me using decision analysis could mean compromising my treatment and my life, so Terry and I agreed to persist.

Shortly before noon, Sandra came in, did the physical exam, announced that my lumps were clearly smaller and that most that she remembered had disappeared completely, and said that she was optimistic that the treatment was working. All that was good news, and telling it first was probably sensible, given Terry's and my level of irritation. "But where were you this morning?" Terry asked. "We had a staff meeting I couldn't get out of," Sandra said, somewhat tentatively, echoing the Fellow. "But we really need to talk about what to do here," I said. "I'm very concerned that we have not had a full discussion about the pros and cons of all the various long-term treatment options, and I really need it!" "Well, maybe we can try to squeeze it in next time," Sandra said without committing to anything definite.

I took another tack: "You have to eat sometime; can we take you to dinner and discuss it then so it doesn't interfere with your busy day?" "Well, I travel half the time, to meetings and other things, you know, like you do." "Like I *did* before these treatments left me immune-compromised," I corrected. "Okay," she said. "I promise to stay late after clinic three weeks from today so we can talk." "Fine. When should we get here?" "Clinic ends at 6:00 p.m., so come in for your appointment late that afternoon, and just stick around afterwards." "Agreed," I said. "Draw a flow chart of what's on your mind so we can talk about it," Sandra suggested. "Great, we'll do that."

We left, Terry still angry that the doctors had blown off the appointment without even warning us. "It's passive-aggressive behavior, and that's no way for doctors to be," she said. "They're the best there is," I reminded her. "They're busier than all heck, they're used to a hierarchical system, and they're not accustomed to dealing with patients from hell. We'll just be persistent, and it'll work out." She calmed down, perhaps having undergone an out-of-body experience herself, and she agreed that we'd try once again to have a frank and open discussion with the doctors about the pros and cons of various approaches and long-term treatment options.

Asking for Answers and Attention

My single word of advice to patients and advocates in this situation is: persevere. When you or someone you know has a dread disease, you deserve to have your questions answered and your fears addressed, but it might take some work. Once you have received your diagnosis, and perhaps a prognosis, begin by researching your disease and jotting down a list of questions and concerns you have about your condition and treatment. As time passes, you may add to or subtract from the list as necessary—yet another example of Bayesian updating.

If there comes a point when you need to schedule a meeting of your own, mull it over or discuss it with your advocate to decide on the best course of action, and then approach your medical team with your request. Remember that your doctors are merely mortals, albeit busy ones, and your concerns should be theirs. It is possible to approach them in a polite-yet-firm manner, and I imagine you'll be surprised at your own courage under fire. When your life is on the line, there's no room for backing down or settling for second best.

Try to decide whether the doctor who is treating you for your disease or other specialists—like Ron Levy and others, in my case—will be able to answer your questions most effectively. If you think you need the help of someone other than your doctor, I suggest you look on the Web and see who else at your hospital or medical institute is well versed in your disease or in a process that might be helpful in treating it, and then expand your search to other hospitals and medical institutions. Once you have found a few people you think can help you, familiarize yourself with their work and learn about their current projects by reading whatever material is available on and by them. When you decide to contact them, e-mail tends to be an excellent mode of communication, as phone messages seem to get lost in the fray more often. E-mail will give you the chance to give in-depth details on your condition and ask clear and concise questions of the specialist.

Showing that you are knowledgeable about your disease and the work of the specialist you are contacting and asking targeted questions will likely help you get his or her attention. In the real world, alas, it also doesn't hurt to have some sort of inside connection. When contacting Ron Levy, I brought up his daughter, Karen, who had been a student in one of my courses. I mentioned that I had actually met Ron at the celebration we held for Karen when we awarded her a prize for her superb thesis. Don't be afraid to ask your friends, neighbors, and family members if they know anything about the specialists you are trying to contact. It is likely that some of them have experience with dread diseases, either directly or through another friend or loved one, and you never know who in the medical world they may know. Ask your primary care doctor, if you have one, if he or she is acquainted with any of these specialists or any other specialists who could help you. If you are attending a support group for your disease, ask other members whom they know in the medical world. If you don't think you have any connections, don't be discouraged. The medical community—especially for uncommon diseases—is smaller than you think, and it's likely that you'll be able to make one.

A Frank and Open Discussion

After three weeks and much reservation about whether we'd get our hourlong session with Sandra, Terry and I headed back to the hospital. I got my CT scan in the morning, went in to see Sandra that afternoon, and got all my lumps felt. "Hard to find any lumps on you," she said excitedly. "The Fellow couldn't either! I really think we'll get a good CT scan result and that the treatments are working well." This was no doubt a much less stressful meeting than the previous one, and Terry and I both felt as if a huge weight had been lifted off our chests. Sandra told us to come back in a few hours, when she would be finished with clinic, and we could—at last!—have our decision analysis chat.

We went back at 6:00 p.m., and, slowly but surely, the last of the patients dribbled out of Oncology Day Care, as did the nurses, the members of the scheduling staff, who spent their days busily typing away at their computer terminals, and the blood-draw team. Terry and I sat in one of the standard examination rooms, and although we could see docs coming and going, looking at charts and X-rays and conversing among themselves, there was no sign of Sandra. I looked at Terry and thought, *This can't happen twice, not after she promised.* Terry knew what was going through my mind, and she looked at me doubtfully. "I would be a completely lousy judge of character if I thought she would do that," I said, and I just had faith that she'd show up. But by 7:30 p.m., even I was beginning to lose hope.

Finally, about ten minutes later, an exhausted Sandra arrived, sat down, and apologized for being late. "It's been a very hard day—many difficult cases and many consultations. Sorry to be so long." "We really appreciate your coming to do this," I said. "I have formulated ten questions rather than a decision flow chart." It turned out Terry had drafted a decision analytic flow chart that we also discussed later on, which appears on page 99. "Okay, let's talk about them," she said.

By that time, I was no longer in denial about needing a bone marrow transplant, and I deduced from Sandra's previous comments that I was going to need radiation treatment as well, although I still wasn't sure why. "Radiation can induce all kinds of trouble, so why is it worth it, particularly if you think the CT scan is going to show that I'm in remission?" "You already told me," she said, "that just because a CT scan determines that you're in remis-

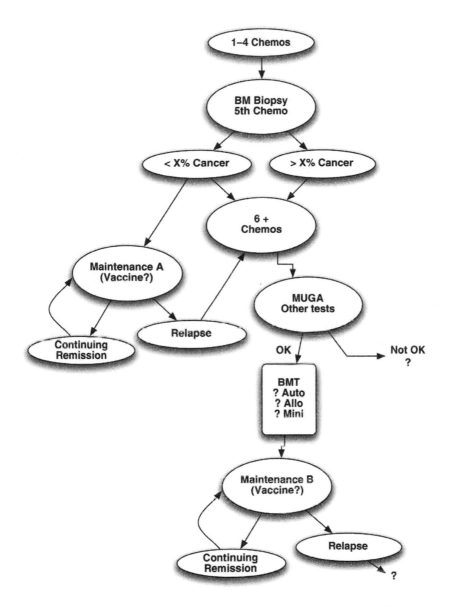

sion, it's not an indication that you have no cancer cells left in your body, and since you have such a sneaky disease, we have to hit it with everything in the arsenal." "What about the side effects of the radiation?" "You haven't read that on the Web yet?" "Well yeah, we have, and it doesn't sound like too much fun." "It's tolerable. Not pleasant, but tolerable." "But why do I need full-body radiation? Why not just irradiate my lymph node system? I don't like the idea of you guys zapping my brain." "It's only 1,300 rads,"[4] she said. "1,300 rads!?!" I exclaimed. "That's almost two and a half lethal doses!"

I remembered from my days of studying nuclear winter in the 1980s that 500 rads would kill at least half the people exposed to it—a measure termed LD50: lethal dose, 50 percent. Sandra tried to comfort me by telling me that people with brain tumors get 5,000 rads to their heads. She was nearly certain that 1,300 would not affect my thinking. She explained that the radiation was done in fractionated form. It would be divided into two or three doses a day over four and a half days, so I'd never be getting more than about 150 rads at any one time. This would allow some of my benign fast-growing cells to recover a little bit but wouldn't cause my cancer to come back too much; we'd get almost the same cancer kill rate as we would if we administered the whole 1,300 rads at once. Also, I'd be under the care of the hospital and receiving many transfusions afterward, rather than being forced to fend for myself with a collapsed immune system, as would be the fate of millions in the case of nuclear war.

I asked, "Are you sure this isn't going to affect my memory or my reasoning skills?" "Even if you lost a few IQ points, you wouldn't know the difference," she joked. "None of my patients have had any trouble returning to their normal ways of life afterward, and none have said that they had any detectable loss of brain power." "But why irradiate my head?" She explained once again that my lymphoma could be hiding out in a node behind my eyeball, and we just had to have an alternative kill mechanism if we wanted a reasonably high probability of a long remission. Sandra still wouldn't use the "C" word, and we guessed that "cure" did not exist in her vocabulary, given the experiences she'd had with these nasty diseases.

"What about the mucositis?"[5] Terry asked. "The mucositis *will* be very nasty," Sandra said, "as the mucous membranes from the bottom of your colon to the top of your throat will certainly undergo serious trauma, but we have plenty of analgesics and other methods for dealing with that. Typically, the mucositis only lasts a few weeks, and the benefits of radiation are well worth the pain." "What about the probability that the radiation will induce leukemia?" I asked worriedly. "It's something on the order of 5 to 7 percent," she said. I could feel the color drain out of my face. "So not only would I have the mucositis, but I'd have a 5 to 7 percent chance of leukemia?" I was beginning to wonder if this was worth it. "Yeah, that's what the data show." "When does this leukemia manifest itself?" "It usually doesn't appear until several years after the radiation." "Is it treatable?" "Yes, by another bone marrow transplant. But don't worry about it; it's not an immediate side effect, and it isn't very common. New treatments are being discovered all the time, and by the time you developed leukemia, the treatments would be more effective, less painful, and shorter in duration." *Am I supposed to find this comforting?* I wondered.

"Well, in order to do a true decision analysis," I said, "I'd like to weigh the benefits and costs of the radiation in terms of what it does for my health." "Okay," she said, "ask away." "Sandra, suppose there are 100 patients like me with my strength, my condition, and my disease. How many of them do you think would get radiation-induced leukemia several years from now?" I asked the question as if it were a frequency—that is, how many out of 100 rather than focusing only on my case—because cognitive psychology has shown that when people are asked to give a probabilistic estimate for a *single* event, they tend to be overconfident and make an inaccurate estimate, but when asked questions posed as frequencies, their answers are much more accurate. "Like I said, probably something like five to seven of them," Sandra responded. "Now, how many of those patients would still be in remission four years after their treatment ended if they didn't undergo radiation compared with those who did?" "I told you, I can't give you precise numbers," she said, feeling uncomfortable with my subjective analysis. "Just tell me what your intuition is. How many out of 100?" "Well, probably more than fifty would still be in remission after four years if they had the *full* treatment, including radiation. Without full treatment, the number might only be about thirty." "So are you saying that you think full treatment would increase the probability of getting rid of my lymphoma by two-thirds [from 30 percent to 50 percent]?" She nodded.

"Well," I said, "I have the lymphoma now, and that's what we need to worry about fighting. If I'm among the 5 to 7 percent who develop leukemia, which would be delayed by several years, there would be a treatment for it, and by that time it would be very good. And even now, the treatment for the leukemia—an allo bone marrow transplant—is the same treatment I'd have to endure if I lost remission on the cancer I have. Does that sound right?" "That's a good summary." "Then let's do the radiation. I sure didn't want it coming in here, but I'm convinced now that the odds are definitely in favor of doing it." "I agree," she said. "In addition, if we treat you less aggressively by experimenting with maintenance therapy rather than going ahead with the bone marrow transplant and radiation and you lose remission, it'll be much more difficult to achieve a second remission, not to mention that you'll be older and therefore more vulnerable to the treatments and side effects than you are now." That confirmed what I was already beginning to believe.

Terry and I agreed that we'd opt for the whole-body radiation, and Sandra nodded approvingly. "There's one more benefit, too," she said. "People who don't do the radiation are given another round of chemo at the time of the bone marrow transplant, and that one is notorious for weakening the immune system to the point that fungal lung infections occur more often." "Are fungal lung infections serious?" I asked. "They can be," she said. "In fact, with all the construction going on around Stanford and all the dust in the air, it's probably a good idea for you to start wearing a mask when you're walking around campus." I thought back to biking right through the cloud of construction dust when my neutrophil count was below 200, and I realized once again how lucky I was that I didn't have a brush with death right then.

I couldn't conceal any longer that I'd been in touch with Ron Levy without consulting Sandra first: "I sent Ron Levy an e-mail about our discussion of maintenance therapy." "I know," she said, "and I agree that when the time comes, we can talk about it." "The Fellow says there's no frequency data and we shouldn't even think about it, but my intuition tells me that it isn't frequency data that we need but process knowledge. We need to understand how various cancer agents and treatments work on cells, not simply whether or not we've got historical data." "I agree with that," said Sandra, "but it does make me uncomfortable not having any clear data. I certainly think that if it still looks like we need some sort of maintenance therapy after the bone marrow transplant and radiation, we ought to do it. I'd be willing to talk about that in the future."

Distinguishing Frequency Data from Process Knowledge

In dealing with your dread disease, you or an advocate will learn quickly to distinguish between frequency data and "process knowledge," which is just what it sounds like: knowledge about a process—in this case, what treatments do and how the body reacts. As previously mentioned, in treating dread diseases, doctors have come to rely on frequency data, which basically consist of large sets of historical results from clinical trials that were conducted on hundreds, or even thousands, of patients, some who got the medicine, device, or procedure being tested, others who got placebos. Such data allow for statistical analysis and observations on what course of action is best for the "average" patient. You may also hear frequency data being referred to as statistical, objective, empirical, or clinical trials data. Many in the medical community simply refer to the use of frequency data as "evidence-based medicine." Most standard protocols at state-of-the-art hospitals are based on frequency data, and most doctors prefer to use them, to avoid uncertainties in outcomes as well as to avoid lawsuits. (See the Web site of the Centre for Evidence-Based Medicine [http://www.cebm.utoronto.ca], or do a Web search for "evidence-based medicine" and you'll get thousands of hits. Searching for information on process knowledge in medicine yields little. I did a search of the above Web site for the words "Bayesian" and "subjective," and guess what? I did not get a single hit, implying that the full tool kit of decision science may not yet be adequately applied to medicine.)

Clinical trials data are an excellent starting point in treating many diseases. I'd rather have a doctor err on the side of using conservative clinical trials data than on his or her experience with one or two patients, which may border on quackery. But I am against relying *only* on clinical trials data, especially for diseases for which data are minimal. There are many ways to gather evidence, and clinical trials are an important one, but not the only one—and sometimes not the best one. In addition, as I argue throughout this book, even when clinical trials data show what is best for the "average" patient, that may not be best for you. What if you have very different sensitivities to medicine or severity of illness than the "average" patient? Then your doctor could do individualized tests to better describe your condition (like mine did to type and stage my cancer). In addition, your doctors should know how various treatments—both mainstream and not—work, how treatments for diseases similar to yours might work for you, what treatments are unlikely to be effective, and how your overall health could be affected. Situations in which process knowledge is the best knowledge available are ideal for the use of the Bayesian updating discussed earlier. This, too, is "evidence-based medicine," even if many doctors don't yet recognize that it is every bit as scientific as traditional clinical trials.

Medical schools train future doctors in decision analysis, and this is definitely a step in the right direction, as it will help to expand the definition of "evidence-based" medicine in the future. However, the application of many powerful decision-analysis techniques hasn't penetrated the practice of medicine to the extent necessary. It needs to spread from a few practitioners and the theoretical classroom level to the practical hospital level, and soon, since it could be an important supplement to clinical trials—when they are available. A broader array of decision-analytic methods is likely to significantly improve patient care.

To jump-start the use of process knowledge in your own case, talk to your doctors to determine how much you resemble the statistically average patient depicted in the results of clinical trials. Find out how much frequency data directly applicable to you and your condition are available. If the answer is "not enough," ask about incorporating process knowledge into your treatment regimen. It may be smart to start by looking at treatments for diseases similar to yours but that are better understood and asking your doctors whether something similar might work for you. Remember the risk equation: risk equals what can happen multiplied by the odds of it happening. Explore a wide range of treatment outcomes—good and bad—and the probabilities associated with them, and you will gain great understanding of the risks and benefits of options available to you.

—|—

Our decision analysis meeting continued, with my asking Sandra what the real costs would be of maintenance therapy with Rituxan. I mentioned that the financial costs—my medical bills showed that Rituxan was $15,000 per bottle—were irrelevant; I'd find some way to pay for it if the insurance company wouldn't. What I needed to know was the cost-benefit calculation *in the units of my health*. Even if there were only a 20 percent chance that I had undetectable rogue cancer cells remaining after the transplant (which is called minimal residual disease, or MRD), that seemed to be a risk large enough to justify maintenance therapy. "Using Rituxan won't be as dangerous as the CHOP protocol, will it?" I asked Sandra. "It doesn't carry the same risks of heart and lung problems, nerve damage, and other costs to my body, right?" "Well, there may be a small risk of B cells not receptive to the monoclonal antibody treatment you received being boosted," she worried out loud. "But if I had a rare B cell without a CD-20 receptor, meaning the monoclonal antibody wouldn't stick to it, it wouldn't be like antibiotic resistance to bacteria, which can evolve [whereas cancer is just a clone], would it?" "Probably not," she said, "but we can't view it as a zero risk. That is a potential cost to take into consideration when deciding on Rituxan maintenance therapy."

I didn't know enough microbiology to evaluate whether this risk—the possibility of some of my B cells mutating so that they were no longer CD-20 receptive and could not be treated with Rituxan—was a 1 percent risk or a 20 percent risk. There was too little information. Deep uncertainty did indeed mark this decision analysis—and unlike the academic exercises I do with my students for long-term climate change risks and policy options, my life was hanging on this cost-benefit balance, and it was scary to be so unsure of the odds. I rationalized that if maintenance therapy would significantly reduce an estimated 20 percent chance of my having residual cancer, and my risk of dying from the Rituxan maintenance therapy was much less than 20 percent, then simply doing the maintenance therapy seemed a wise precaution. This is precisely the type of decision-analysis calculation that needs to penetrate medicine and become standard practice. However, I did understand that we were wandering into uncharted territory when considering maintenance therapy with Rituxan; there was no telling it would work and no previous data that might help us develop a treatment plan.

I made a second request: "I don't want my future to hinge on the results of a CT scan. If a CT scan won't see my cancer until there are hundreds of millions of malignant cells running rampant in my body, then why don't I get a PCR so that I can know if I have even a few?" Sandra frowned. "PCR is an experimental technique that has barely been used on lymphoma patients. Even if we did it, we wouldn't know exactly how to interpret the results, since we'd have nothing to compare them to."

"Well, I'd at least like to have my stem cell fluid PCR'ed before it is inserted back into my body in the bone marrow transplant, because isn't it possible that there could be rogue cancer cells left in there, and I'd get the whole disease all over again?"[6] "We have very good techniques for purging the stem cells," she said, but she did not deny that PCR would improve my chance of getting cancer-free stem cell fluid reinjected. That reminded me of something else I'd read: "We understand from Rick Murdock's book on his cancer experience, *Patient Number One*, that your husband was involved in the creation of a blood-cleansing machine, the most recent version now being called the Isolex 300i, and the author claims it helped save his life."[7] "Yes, that was Richard Miller, my husband," Sandra said, impressed that we'd picked up on that detail but also leery of what my next outrageous suggestion would be. "I gather that the Isolex 300i is supposed to be ten times more effective at cleaning stem cells than the old machine," I said excitedly. "The machine isn't approved by the FDA [Food and Drug Administration] in the United States," Sandra countered. "I know, but why couldn't I be put on a research protocol so we could use the Isolex on my stem cells?"

Sandra still seemed skeptical, but Terry and I continued to work on her. "The data collected from a series of experiments in Europe seem to show that it's quite successful," Terry said. "I've heard something about that," Sandra said. "Well, we thought this might help," Terry said, handing her the twenty-page report on the European results. She had downloaded it from the Web for our meeting. "Can I keep this?" Sandra asked. "Of course." "All we want is the best possible treatment for me and all your patients," I begged. "We've been thinking about this already, but it's not easy to change procedures," she replied. "Let me look into this and give it some thought."

We all glanced at our watches. It was five minutes past 9:00. Terry and I left, feeling satisfied that our points had been made and heard. The meeting marked a sea change in our relationship with Sandra. A mutual respect developed between us, and I felt like we had finally transcended the traditional doctor-patient hierarchy. Not only was Sandra more open to our ideas and less impatient with our questions from then on, but, as I'll discuss later, changes were made to the protocol based on her thoughtful examination of some of the issues we raised. Obviously, she had to convince those within her own bureaucracy to agree to these protocol exceptions, and we are still grateful to her for going to battle behind the scenes largely on the basis of the decision-analysis approach I advocate in this book.

On our way home Terry said, "You were right to stay with Sandra. She really is spectacular, knows the field, and when she finally had the time, she listened with an open mind." I happily agreed, though I still had underlying concerns about my stem cell fluid to be reinjected in the transplant containing rogue cancer cells and about the side effects of two and a half lethal doses of radiation, which loomed in my near future.

7 | What's So Special About Fifty-Five?

How Full Is "Full Remission"?

"You're in full remission after only three chemos; it's a remarkable achievement!" Sandra told me as I came in for my fourth chemo session. "I gathered from your last physical exam that your lymph nodes were shrinking, but the CT scan shows you as fully normal." "That's wonderful news," I said, trying to echo her degree of excitement but remembering that many, many cancer cells must be present before a CT scan detects the disease. "But what's the probability that there are still cancer cells hiding somewhere?" "You're right to have some doubts," Sandra said, "and that's why we need to do a bone marrow biopsy today, to be sure the remission is as strong as the CT scan suggests and to help determine how to proceed with the bone marrow transplant."

"Well, if the bone marrow biopsy shows full remission too, does that mean I don't need the bone marrow transplant?" I asked hopefully, but fully expecting a rebuff. "No, as I've said, this is a sneaky disease, and even if the biopsy results are excellent, we have to go ahead with the transplant. That will give you the best chances for a long remission. We want the bone marrow biopsy to show a very low cancer cell count, as that will give us the highest probability of an effective transplant. Patients at your stage whose biopsies show significant amounts of cancer in their bone marrow don't usually have the best prognoses, even after they've had bone marrow transplants. I strongly believe the bone marrow transplant is necessary to deal with this difficult disease you have, Steve."

I conceded and took my usual position on my stomach on the little exam table. Terry took her place against the wall and grabbed my hand. I still decided it was best not to look at the needle that would soon be drilling through my bone. Sandra's Fellow entered the room and, seeing that I was in position, said, "You know the drill." I almost said, "Good pun," but I wasn't feeling funny at the time. No matter how much of a veteran one is at bone marrow biopsies—and this was, after all, my third—the anxiety is still pretty high because the pain is a type to which one could never grow accustomed, which guarantees a less-than-pleasant ten minutes. Also, after the physical pain, I would have to suffer through the psychological pain of waiting weeks for the results, hoping that my remission would be confirmed at the higher level of accuracy that the examination of bone marrow fluid provides.

The bone marrow biopsy went about as expected, maybe not quite as painful as the first round, perhaps because I knew what to expect. This time the first extraction of fluid and sample was adequate, so the Fellow didn't have to drill me twice. "I think the results will be much better than last time," he predicted, "given how fantastic the CT scan was three weeks ago." "I sure hope so," I said, trying to ignore the ache in my hip.

Sandra returned shortly after the bone marrow biopsy and asked, "How are you feeling after your first three chemos?" "Pretty good, other than the nausea I get in the first few days after the chemo and the mood-altering effects of the prednisone 'taper'." Terry smiled, remembering the incident in the car a few weeks back, but she kept quiet. I went on: "I've noticed lately that my temperature regulation is off, too, and I yo-yo between feeling hot and cold. I'm just lacking some of my normal get-up-and-go." "Are you still teaching, writing, giving lectures?" Sandra asked. "Of course! I couldn't tolerate this without being able to live a little and feel productive," I said. Sandra raised her eyebrows. "Many people undergoing what you are couldn't even begin to contemplate doing all that, so I'd say that not only have your treatments been very effective, but you're experiencing relatively few side effects." I smiled appreciatively but already felt the anxiety of waiting for the bone marrow biopsy results descend.

Terry and I went upstairs for my fourth round of chemo, and this time I was able to soak up the 750-milliliter upside-down wine bottle of Rituxan in only a few hours. The nurses had been correct—the horrible side effects were only a first-time event, and I took in the Rituxan at a rate of 200 milliliters or more per hour. The nurses, outfitted in rubber gloves to be certain that their skin wouldn't be eaten alive if the vesicant chemos (which would be injected after the Rituxan) splattered on them, removed the Rituxan bottle and began to attach the next vile potion. Despite the chain mail suit imposed on me by the Benadryl drip, I watched all the connections of the tubes running from the chemo solutions to my arm like a hawk. Between the first and the second vesicants, I noticed a little bit of wetness at one of the junctures. I pointed this out to the nurse, who said, "Amazing you could see that. You're right, that needs to be fixed." She wiped off the slight drip and then changed all of the tubes, making the fittings really tight. I then got my injection of vincristine, followed by the small bag of Cytoxan, and before it was even dark outside, I was heading home with Terry, the Benadryl haze just starting to lift and the Compazine beginning to quash my nausea.

—| |—

The three weeks leading up to my fifth chemo session and my appointment with Sandra went by fairly quickly. The prime symptom of the chemotherapy was now exhaustion rather than nausea, so I didn't spend the interim period feeling completely miserable—just tired. I have to admit, though, that my foreboding over both the bone marrow biopsy results and the impending bone marrow transplant, which was to happen in six weeks, was steadily escalating.

Forty Percent to Zero in Twelve Weeks?

When my fifth chemo appointment finally rolled around, I went in for my one-hour appointment with Sandra, and after a few minutes—not the usual few hours' wait—the Fellow came bounding in, beaming, and said, "This is the most remarkable thing I've seen in a long time!" "What?" I inquired. "Your bone marrow biopsy shows none, zero, cancer, and that's absolutely amazing considering the first one, twelve weeks ago, showed that 40 percent of the cells in your marrow were cancer." Instead of celebrating, I said, "What? Forty percent cancer?" "Yes." "Why didn't you tell us that earlier?" I fumed. "What would you have done with the information?" he asked. "It wouldn't have changed anything we did, and it would've made you worry even more. Now you should absolutely celebrate this fabulous news."

The usual dark cloud rose in my left brain. "But how do you know the count is actually zero?" I asked the Fellow. He explained that that was what the pathology report had said. My bone marrow fluid was observed under a microscope, and no cancer cells were found, whereas the results of my previous bone marrow biopsy showed that about 40 percent of my fluid was made up of cancer cells. If we hadn't caught the lymphoma then, all of my marrow could have been filled up with cancer cells in a few short months. I knew what that meant: bad news for the life insurance company.

Still doggedly skeptical, I posed the question about my cancer cell count a bit differently: "Are you completely confident it's zero? I presume you receive a pathology report written by a human being, who uses his or her bare eyes to look through a microscope at a slide with a drop of bone marrow fluid on it." "Yes, and it's fabulous news that this human being could not see any cancer cells. It's one of the best results I've ever seen in a cancer patient after only four chemos. It bodes very well for the success of the bone marrow transplant." *Hmmm, I thought to myself, he's already guessed that I was going to ask why I need a bone marrow transplant if I have zero cancer.*

But in truth, I didn't believe that we really knew whether I had zero cancer or not, so I pressed on. "How many cells are in a drop of bone-marrow fluid on a glass slide?" I asked. "I don't know. Quite a lot." "Millions?" "Probably." I wanted to know how a human being spending, say, five minutes viewing my bone marrow slide could possibly be 100 percent accurate. If only a very small percentage of mantle cell lymphoma cells were buried in those millions of normal cells—and thank God they were mostly normal—how would they ever be seen? (It was a cancer equivalent of "finding Waldo" in a throng of thousands, and the mantle cell Waldo wouldn't be wearing red and white stripes!) If I did have some cancer cells remaining, yet they weren't seen in the slide, we'd be living under the illusion that I was cured, at the same time that my cancer cells could be doubling every month, and I'd be back to having 40 percent of my marrow filled with cancer in a year or two. "I want an absolute zero, not an eyeball zero, which probably gives us a 50 percent chance that it isn't zero." The Fellow, now on to my stubbornness, knew that I was hinting at wanting PCR again. "PCR is still an experimental technique for this cancer, and it would be hard for us to interpret the results," he said, heading for the door, and I understood that he had a host of other, very sick patients to deal with. "Discuss it with Sandra," I requested. "I certainly will."

About an hour later, Sandra came in with a big smile. "You were told the great news?" "Yes," Terry and I said simultaneously. "But Sandra, I still wonder whether it's a hard zero." "I figured you would." Sandra confirmed that it was impossible to verify the zero count given the technique used to analyze the samples taken in the bone marrow biopsy. She explained that this uncertainty was one of the reasons that she felt it was so important that I go through with the bone marrow transplant. We had worked very hard to knock out any rogue cells that were hiding anywhere: in my bone marrow, in a random lymph node, or, most worrying, behind one of my eyeballs on the other side of the blood-brain barrier—the spot we had discussed during our decision analysis three weeks earlier, when we decided that the side effects and other risks of a Hiroshima-dose of whole-body radiation were worth it.

Isolex Success!

"I have more good news for you," Sandra said. "I reviewed the downloads you gave me on the Isolex 300i machine, checked with a number of people I know, discussed it with the department, and the machine has been ordered. I think you'll end up being the third or fourth patient in this hospital whose blood will be purified by that machine when you get your stem cells removed in late December." Terry and I looked at each other, awestruck, feeling rather proud that we had not only helped modify the protocol in a way that, given our knowledge at the time, seemed most likely to improve my odds, but that other patients were going to benefit from it as well. Sandra's willingness to listen earnestly to our concerns and look into new treatment options when they seemed to have potential showed the benefits of our dialogue. I told Sandra how much we appreciated her efforts. I imagine it took a significant personal intervention on her part, especially in the face of the committee that approves new treatments and equipment investments. She never let on as to whether accomplishing that purchase was an ordeal for her.

I knew that the Isolex 300i machine was relatively inexpensive, probably less than $100,000, which is below the noise level in a hospital, but when I found out it would take an office, two technicians, and a Ph.D. scientist to run the machine, it was clear that the hospital was making a nontrivial investment. Sandra and her colleagues must have been convinced that the machine's potential to increase the precision and efficacy of the stem cell cleaning was well worth experimentation, even if there were no extensive data sets to prove it.

I thanked Sandra again, and she replied that it was nothing and that modernization was necessary, even at Stanford: "We have to start somewhere in seeing how the Isolex works and interpreting the results. Hopefully, we can add this to our treatment arsenal."

Since the time of our decision analysis talk with Sandra, the FDA had approved the use of the Isolex machine for cleaning stem cells, but it was still an experimental technique, so I would have to sign up under a research protocol in order to have it used on my stem cells. Of course, signing on to a research protocol meant that I would no longer be a useful patient in Sandra's standard mantle cell lymphoma database. Most of the patients she and her team were following had received CHOP chemotherapy plus Rituxan, the monoclonal antibody, just as I had, but my results would not be comparable because we would also be using the Isolex machine, and the previous twenty or thirty patients had not. It also meant that we wouldn't have any real statistics against which we could compare my results, so we would have to use process knowledge to interpret them.

Although I'd been granted my wish of getting to use the Isolex, I would have to contend with an uncomfortable degree of deep uncertainty about what the results meant for the likelihood of remission. There were precious little data anywhere about the use of the Isolex machine on patients treated with something similar to the Stanford protocol of CHOP plus Rituxan. *The research disease I've got is certainly testing my belief in decision analysis*, I thought to myself, but I was very pleased that someone significant (Sandra) was listening.

The "Fifty-five and Under" Rule

The good news couldn't last forever. After telling us about the Isolex, Sandra said, "There is one aspect of our decision analysis discussion that I will have to retract." Her brow wrinkled in a way that made me nervous. "What's that?" "Whole-body radiation. You can't get it." "What?" I exclaimed. I couldn't believe that she'd reversed her earlier opinion, especially after our analysis of all the pros and cons led us to decide that it was the best possible option. I asked if there were new data suggesting that our discussion of the risks and benefits of radiation was off by some large factor, and Sandra said it was nothing of the sort. Rather, it was another "medicine by the numbers" problem: The protocol stipulated that nobody over fifty-five years old could receive such a large dose of whole-body radiation. I was fifty-six, so Sandra said I didn't qualify. "Is there really a difference between being fifty-five and fifty-six years old?" I asked incredulously, my voice rising. "The cutoff seems completely arbitrary." "Yes, it's arbitrary," Sandra explained, "but it's a threshold that's been established by doctors based on the side effects of the radiation."

My left brain then took over the conversation. I asked Sandra what it was that correlated with age and radiation that wouldn't make the benefits of the extra kill power from the radiation worth the risk. Her answer was heart and lung damage, not inconsequential side effects. It was a legitimate concern, but I persisted. I figured the threshold was based on the health of the "average" patient, and that age fifty-five was the cutoff point at which, on average, younger patients did better with the treatment and older patients did worse. Sandra agreed. I also figured that there must be a lot of variation among patients, as very few were actually "average." There were probably fifty-year-old patients who were weaker than average and could be dangerously harmed by radiation, whereas there were probably other patients near sixty who were stronger than average and could tolerate radiation rather well. Sandra agreed once again. I went in for the kill: "So, let's do the tests. Let's find out whether my heart and lung conditions are above or below age normal and allow that piece of information to drive the decision." "It's not in the protocol," Sandra said. "I'll pay for the tests myself." "You can't," she said, reminding me of my earlier experience with Neupogen and protocols, which showed that, in hospitals, there are limits to what a patient's money can buy. "Then write me an order for the tests that are needed. I'll do them at another hospital, and I'll have them send you the results."

Sandra didn't say anything but started writing something down on a yellow slip of paper, the same paper she used to order CT scans and other tests for me. She said, "Okay, I agree with your logic. Here are orders to get an arterial blood test for lung function and a MUGA[1] heart scan for ejection fraction, which will tell us whether your age or the chemos you've had thus far have left you unfit for radiation." I thanked her again, appreciating her open-mindedness and that she was again resorting to decision analysis. In fact, I had a sneaking suspicion that Sandra had probably played out this entire scenario in her head before she even walked in, went through the perfunctory process of informing me of the rules during our actual discussion, fully knowing I'd fight it, and then used her clout in the hospital to override the rules. It was becoming increasingly evident that Sandra really did buy into decision analysis and concurred with Terry and me that following protocols based on standardized measures, such as the age of the "average" patient, was not necessarily the best way to treat any one individual—hence the order for the tests.

The heart and lung tests would tell us whether I was better or worse than age normal and essentially determine whether I got whole-body radiation or not. I suspected that my heart and lungs were in excellent condition, because the previous August, when 40 percent of my marrow was dominated by cancer, I had no symptoms other than lymph node enlargement and no loss of energy at all; I felt like a perfectly normal person. But even if my heart and lungs were in great shape, I was confronted by a nasty Catch-22: If I "lost" and was below age normal, it meant that my heart and lungs were already weak and I would not be eligible for radiation, which would increase my chances of a relapse. If I "won," I would get a Hiroshima-dose of radiation, accompanied by horrible side effects, including the risk of cataracts and leukemia. Neither option was thrilling. I felt fatalistic and thought, *I already had to make the choice about radiation once, and I sure don't want to have to revisit it, so I'll just let the tests decide.*

Fight or Flight?

In dealing with a dread disease, it is impossible for a patient or his or her advocate to fight every single battle over treatment, but there is a way to decide when to fight and when to take flight. First and foremost, if something comes up—as the possibility of not being able to get radiation therapy did for me—that could dramatically affect your outcome, it is well worth a fight. Don't be afraid to ask to have a protocol overridden or to ask whether alternative solutions are available. If such a problem seems to have many solutions, great, but if not, don't give up; it may still be worth pursuing, because your advocate and medical team may have yet more ideas. When problems arise that most likely won't affect your long-term health, you must pick your battles. Again, if you see a simple solution to the problem, bring it up. I did that later on for things like the timing of Neupogen shots and morphine drips and other small details of my treatment that didn't have an impact on my outcome but improved my quality of life. For other problems—like my complaint about not being able to get the results of tests taken at my previous appointment until the next appointment, discussed below—the energy it takes and the goodwill you use up may not be worth the struggle. Just shrug it off and learn to wait.

Waiting . . . and Waiting . . . and Waiting . . .

The last week of the three-week wait between my chemo treatments was always incredibly stressful, even though it was the week I felt most normal, since my white counts were back up, my liver had detoxified the chemo chemicals, and I could go out to eat and even drink some wine. The hard part, it turned out, was dealing with the anxiety that built up ahead of my next appointment with Sandra and the Fellow, where I would find out the results of tests taken during the previous appointment or in the interim, results I wished could have just been sent to me in an e-mail as soon as they were available—undoubtedly only a few days after I took them. Rather, Terry and I went through the agony of waiting until our scheduled appointment to get the latest scoop on the probabilities of life or death. Although I'd become used to the waiting, I couldn't control the apprehension that came with it; I could sense it spilling over into every aspect of my daily life, usually manifested as a shortness of patience on issues having nothing to do with my cancer. I knew it couldn't be a symptom of the prednisone withdrawal, since that occurred in the first week after chemo, so I was sure it was just a result of the frustration I felt about having to wait for answers of grave importance, and answers that I probably could have been told much earlier if the hospital's procedures allowed for it. But apparently they didn't. I knew that part of this logic was not only that hospitals wanted doctors to spend their time treating patients rather than making phone calls and sending e-mails, but also that they believed that only the doctors could properly explain the results to their patients. Giving patients the numbers before an appointment might cause them to misinterpret them and overreact. I agreed that uninterpreted results are not for everyone, but I felt that I was capable of understanding them, especially with resources like the Web and my friends in the medical profession. Having an extra week or two to think over the test results would have given me a chance to formulate even better questions and arguments for my office visits with Sandra, rather than being forced to react and perhaps make decisions on the spot. If I received the results ahead of time, I'd have the chance to hit the Web, the telephone, or e-mail to get up to speed on what it all meant and then have a more productive and focused discussion with Sandra at my next appointment.

Having no control over this aspect of the protocol, and no clear sign that I would ever be able to change it, I just pretended not to worry. Nevertheless, I could feel the tension build as that third week wound down and we approached our Tuesday morning appointment at the Oncology Day Care Center.

—|⊢—

Finally, the interminable wait was over, and we headed to our morning meeting with Sandra, which preceded my fifth chemo treatment. The Fellow entered the room, felt me up perfunctorily, and said, "No need to test you. Between the CT scan and the bone marrow biopsy, we know you don't have any palpable lymphoma. Just one quick check. Nope, you don't have any large nodes in your neck or armpits." Normally, I would be concerned at not having a thorough exam, but this time I was relieved that I didn't get poked and prodded too much when it was completely obvious that the probability of Sandra or the Fellow detecting cancer by poking was well below the probability that a CT scan or bone marrow biopsy would pick it up. Indeed, I appreciated being spared the uncomfortable indignity.

Eventually Sandra came in and agreed that my progress was fabulous. Before I had a chance to ask any questions, she began setting up appointments for me for the bone marrow transplant, which would be taking place in another month or so. She gave us the names of nurses, social workers, radiation oncologists, and others to visit, and we were assured that they would explain the procedure to us from beginning to end: what we'd have to do, how we'd have to do it, why the hospital stay was so long, and when I'd feel like a human being again.

During her abbreviated explanation of the bone marrow transplant, Sandra mentioned that the radiation treatment would take place the week *before* I checked into the hospital. After that, I would get two lethal chemo treatments (megadoses of Cytoxan and another myeloablative drug known as VP-16), and then, because of the chemos, and especially because of the radiation, I would have to stay in isolation in a clean room in the hospital for about three weeks.

I picked up on Sandra's comments on radiation immediately. "So the results of the heart and lung tests were good, then?" "You're way better than age normal, so based on our decision analysis, we should go ahead with the radiation as we originally agreed. I'm glad I was able to get the group [of my colleagues in the oncology department] to see it that way as well." I thanked Sandra for intervening again on my behalf. She smiled sheepishly and continued writing orders for visiting various nurses, doctors, and technicians in the bone marrow unit. These visits were going to keep us busy in the period leading up to my sixth chemo session and for a week or so thereafter.

That reminded me: "Why am I getting a sixth chemo if the bone marrow biopsy shows that my cancer count is so low? The chemos have serious side effects, so it's not worth doing if I don't need it." "Well, we've clearly got your cancer on the run, but if there are a few cells left, as you and I both worry, the more chemo we do, the fewer cells there are likely to be, which increases the chances of an effective bone marrow transplant. One more chemo is fine. You're tolerating them well, and your heart and lungs are still in very good condition, even after four chemos. Let's stay with the plan." I readily agreed.

As we walked out of Sandra's office, I was not thinking very much about the chemo I was about to get upstairs. My cancer thoughts returned to my concern that there could be a few rogue cancer cells left in my stem cell fluid, even after six chemos and the processing of my blood in the Isolex 300i, and we would never know it if we didn't PCR it. Now that I think about it, I did bring that issue back up again with Sandra, but she quickly said the usual: "We wouldn't know how to interpret it." Basically, in a polite way, she said no. I still wasn't convinced, but I had won a number of battles on the way to individualizing my treatments, and I guess I was a little worn out, so I didn't bother to press the matter further. In retrospect, I think I should have been dramatically more aggressive about getting PCR for the stem cell fluid before it was reinjected in the auto transplant.

Coulda, Shoulda

Even a patient from hell will realize retrospectively that there were many other things that could have been done or asked for along the course of treatment. While some aspects of treatment can't be anticipated, others can. To avoid having too many regrets about your own treatment, do all the research you can about your disease. Any information on new and successful treatment protocols or new technology or machinery (like the Isolex) will likely be helpful. Once again, if you're fighting for some treatment option that you think could significantly improve your long-term health, don't back down! It's possible that your doctors, who are highly intelligent but sometimes get stuck in routines dictated by protocols, will come to see things your way, or they may give you good arguments why you are wrong. Then either outcome will be positive and will at least give you peace of mind.

8 | Graduation to the Bone Marrow Unit

I WAS LIGHTHEARTED AND OPTIMISTIC during the time leading up to my sixth chemo session, not only because I felt that my treatment had been relatively successful and my relationship with Sandra was only getting better, but also because the usual anxiety that dominated my being had vanished. There were no test results that I was going to learn about at the sixth chemo, so there was no reason to be nervous in the preceding weeks. Terry and I were just focusing on preparing for the transplant procedure, which included a visit to Stanford Hospital's bone marrow unit.

The (Next) Uphill Climb

On our way to the bone marrow unit, we navigated through the hospital until we saw a large sign on the wall that read "BMT," with an arrow pointing toward the main door. At least it was easy to find. Inside, we were greeted by a rather impressive sight. Patients, about half of whom were completely bald or obviously wearing wigs and about a quarter of whom were wearing face masks with large pink high-efficiency particulate air (HEPA) filter discs, indicating seriously compromised immune systems, were sitting around waiting rooms or inside examination rooms, meeting with nurses, having fluids infused into them, or suffering through the side effects of chemo or posttransplant trauma.

Sometimes, during a long hike, you look up at the mountain looming in front of you and wonder how you'll ever reach the peak. Then you see people coming back down from the top, and you're quite jealous that they've already been there and made it back down to your level safely, when you have so much more up- hill climbing to do. Being the newcomer in the bone marrow unit felt similarly daunting. I knew that there was a long road ahead of me and that most of the patients I was seeing were well ahead of me in the treatment process. Although I might have fantasized about changing places, I knew that some of the posttransplant pa- tients I was seeing probably weren't in full remission before they had their transplants and therefore might not have had nearly as good a prognosis as it appeared I would, given my full remission, high responsiveness to treatment, and the relatively few side ef- fects I had felt up to that point. In addition, none of the patients I saw would have had the Isolex 300i to purge their blood. Sandra had told me that I'd be the third or fourth patient whose blood would be cleansed by it, and that was still another three or four weeks away. So, despite the uphill climb that confronted me, I de- cided that I wasn't willing to trade places with anyone. I'd keep the cancer I had, I'd keep my great treatment results, and I'd defi- nitely keep the relationship I'd established with a terrific doctor.

The Patient Isn't an Idiot After All

My "graduation" from the oncology ward meant that I was now completely under the care of the bone marrow transplant unit; they would take over the scheduling of all my appointments. One of the first big appointments would come a few weeks after my sixth chemo session, when I would have a Hickman catheter in- serted into me, which sounded innocent enough. Once the Hickman catheter was in place, I would not need to have any more IVs stuck into me, and that certainly sounded like a pleasant change from the IV-jabbing experiences I'd had over the previous six months. Curiously, one of the nurses winced every time the Hickman was mentioned, and we wondered why until we learned more about it over subsequent visits.

My sixth chemo session occurred during the school holidays in late December, and afterward my sister Liz and my nieces came to visit. Liz was with us at the hospital when the nurse explained slowly and carefully that the Hickman catheter is a double tube that would be inserted under the skin over my breastbone and then plunged down into my superior vena cava, the large vein that returns oxygen-depleted blood to the heart from the head and arms. This sounded painful, but I was told it was necessary for the autologous bone marrow transplant I was going to have, in which I would get my own stem cells back. Nearly all my blood would be sucked out of one of the tubes (not all at the same time, of course), put into a centrifuge machine that would spin it until the medium- to heavy-weight particles were trapped and removed, and then the amount needed to keep me alive would be injected back into me through the other tube. I was a few weeks away from this process, called apheresis.

The catheter had other benefits, too. It could be used for drawing my blood, infusing chemos, and, later on, the many transfusions of red blood cells and platelets that I was inevitably going to need after the radiation wiped out my natural stem cells' capacity to produce those life-sustaining components of the blood. Often I'd be getting more than one chemical at a time, and the Hickman catheter could accommodate that. Most of the time I'd be connected to saline solution through one tube, to keep my body hydrated, while the other tube would be used to inject some chemical or draw blood for testing.

So the Hickman catheter seemed to be worth the trouble, but I still wondered what was so bad about it that its mention could make a nurse wince. One of the nurses kept returning to the issue of "Hickman hygiene," so I presumed that that was the catch. The nurse explained that the opening in the skin where the Hickman went in could become infected and therefore had to be sterilized twice a day. The tube itself had to be sterilized, too, and we had to be absolutely sure of avoiding the very dangerous possibility of creating a clot while doing so. Since the catheter would be in a place where air could meet blood, a clot could form, and since the catheter was placed directly into my superior vena cava, such a clot could cause a pulmonary embolism.[1] This was no joking matter. We were told that the way to prevent clotting was to inject heparin, an anticoagulant, into the tube right after the cleaning, directly after the saline flush. The heparin would prevent any blood that did come in contact with air that made it into the tube from coagulating.

The complex steps for dealing with the Hickman catheter were truly daunting, and I was glad the nurses were going to be performing this. But then the nurses looked at Terry and asked, "You're the primary caretaker?" "Yes," she said nervously. "Well, did you get everything I said? You'll have to do this for him at home." We were shocked. "I think so," Terry replied, still reeling at the thought of being responsible for my "Hickman hygiene." "I've been writing fast. Can I download the instructions from the Web, too?" "No need. I'll give you a brochure. He'll be home for the first phase of the transplant, which will take several weeks, and he'll have the Hickman for weeks after that, so it'll be up to you to do all the sterilizations and the heparin lock and to be sure that everything is working properly."

I trusted Terry completely, and she was very devoted to caring for me, but we were both nervous about the prospect of doing all the Hickman catheter maintenance on our own. "But how do you prevent the blood from flowing back up the tubes and spilling all over the place, draining me out like the unfortunate character in some Sherlock Holmes mystery?" I wondered.

"Good question," said the nurse. "The Hickman has a lock, which is basically a plastic device that works like the catch on a pump-it-yourself gasoline nozzle. When you squeeze on the trigger, you can push down a bar that catches in various positions, giving deep, medium, or light pressure." She gave us a demonstration. "It's very important that you remember to open this lock when you're cleaning the catheter or injecting fluids, then do the heparin, and then quickly squeeze it closed." "What happens if I accidentally knock the tube open in my sleep?" She spared no details. "You'll wake up in a big puddle, and if that happens, just click the valve closed, call the hospital, and come in immediately. Fortunately, it's very rare." I wasn't comforted. "We'll wrap the entire device in a plastic bag so it won't happen to me no matter what," I said. "You can find your own solution, but just remember that it'll be up to you to take care of your own hygiene." *So, the patient isn't an idiot after all,* I thought to myself. *He's expected to take care of the sterility, the heparin lock, and the procedures with the valve clip on a twice-daily basis himself.*

Being informed that I would need to take care of my own Hickman hygiene made me realize this seeming contradiction. On the one hand, as a patient, I was treated as naïve and incapable of understanding test results without interpretation from a doctor. In the beginning, there were also many doubts as to whether I could effectively participate in discussions about my treatment options. On the other hand, as the case of the Hickman illustrated, when it came to complicated home care, I (along with my wife and caretaker) was assumed to be highly competent. The cynic in me couldn't help but wonder whether the fact that my participation in home care would likely save my insurance company money, whereas my participation in my treatment might not, at least in the short term, drove the differing assumptions about my aptitude. I have no data to back this up, so it is only a speculation, but it's one I can't just dismiss as some paranoid musing, given the experience I had earlier with "earning" Neupogen.

Liz put on a happy face during the Hickman catheter discussion and throughout her visit, resorting to what must be an inherited Schneider family left-brained way of thinking. She joked a lot and enjoyed some excellent wine with us, since I was allowed to indulge a bit more now that I was sufficiently past chemo. I appreciated Liz's company and positive attitude; it was hard to be grumpy around her and my nieces. My spirits were also lifted by an increase in card and e-mail traffic from people congratulating me on my full remission and wishing me luck with my upcoming procedure. It was immensely cheering to get so much support, sometimes from people I hadn't heard from in twenty years. I wondered how everybody knew so much about my condition and later found out that every week, Paul Ehrlich had been circulating an e-mail to a group of friends and colleagues whom we both knew well, giving them the blow-by-blow description of what was going on in my life. Paul's support during my disease came as close to the definition of pure friendship as anything I know.

My New Appendage

In the third week of December 2001, the Hickman catheter day rolled around. I had to go to "interventional radiology" to have it put in. "Interventional radiology?" I had asked Sandra at my appointment in her alternate office in the bone marrow unit. "Yes," she said. "We've found that normal surgeons don't like doing procedures like this and that having highly trained technicians who do basically one thing, like inserting Hickman catheters, is a more effective, less side-effect-ridden way to go. The Hickman catheter technicians fall under the department of interventional radiology." Clearly, the hospital knew what it was doing, so I hardly argued. "They're going to give me Versed, aren't they?" I asked nervously. "I don't know what their protocol is, but let me assure you that they know precisely what they're doing," Sandra advised.

After sitting around the BMT zone with Terry and Liz for about an hour, two orderlies came for me with a gurney. "Why can't I walk? I'm not drugged yet," I said. "Procedure," replied the orderly. "We have to roll you in, but your family can come with you up to the door of the operating room." I reluctantly got onto the gurney, and Terry and Liz walked beside me down the hall and then waved good-bye, saying, "We'll see you in half an hour."

The room was like the operating rooms seen on television, with the addition of some radiology equipment, which I assumed the technicians used to be sure that the catheter was being punched into my superior vena cava and not some other tube in my chest. I met the anesthesiologist and asked her, "I'm getting Versed, right?" "Yes, that's the drug we usually give for these." "I never felt or remembered anything when I was on Versed for my lymph node removal," I said, telling her of my experience of having no recollection of anything between asking Harry Oberhelman to take out a second lymph node and having him say, "Everything went fine. I sent an extra lymph node off to Ron Levy's lab." "So," I continued, "tell me, will I need to be awake for any of this? Will you ask me to move or do something?" "Nope." "Well, give me the maximum amount you're willing to." "Don't worry, you'll get a local and then we'll give you the Versed too. Just be forewarned that most people *do* remember some parts of the procedure, especially the tube being slid under the skin."

I didn't believe it. I thought the anesthesiologist was just trying to make me think that I wouldn't get away scot-free again, but she was right: The surgery wasn't another total amnesia experience. In fact, for the first part of the procedure, I heard the technicians talking, felt them poking me, and certainly felt the local anesthetic being injected, but it wasn't horrible. This was no bone marrow biopsy. Then, in what seemed like only five minutes later, I definitely felt that I was gaining consciousness. I could feel something slithering under my skin, followed by a dull ache. I was conscious enough to say to myself, *That must be the insertion; they did warn me I'd probably feel it.* It didn't seem too bad, though, and the next thing I remember was being wheeled down the hall with Terry and Liz standing over me, and fully waking up and heading back to the BMT unit to recover.

When we got back to the BMT unit, we were all curious as to what the catheter would look like protruding out of my body, so I opened my gown to take a peek at my latest accessory. Two little tubes hung out of my chest on the right side, a few inches above heart level and a few inches below my collarbone. I could feel a hard bump where the tubes went in, which, I had been told, was an O-ring designed to prevent fluid from leaking in and out and to keep the insertion point clean. (In fact, now, four years later, there is still a bump under my skin where the O-ring once was, which I imagine will be with me for life.) The entire catheter was held down against my body with medical tape.

Later in the afternoon, while I was still recovering in the bone marrow transplant unit, the nurses came in, showed Terry the heparin lock procedure, reviewed how we should do it at home, and then showed us how to do the cleaning. "You don't have to worry about cleaning it for the next few days because the tape is on, so you'll only have to do the heparin lock," one nurse said. "We'll have you come back in three days to take off the tape, and then we'll clean the area around the insertion point with alcohol and some other chemicals and apply new tape. Then we'll go through the cleaning procedures with you once more, and from that point forward, you'll be responsible for the cleaning."

Terry had been intently observing and furiously taking notes from the corner of the room. Finally, she spoke: "How can he shower?" She was worried about the impracticality of my having the catheter in while at home, and concerned about how it would affect my quality of life. "Just put the whole thing in a plastic bag, tape it to his chest, and try not to get water in it. Then, perhaps, a good time to clean it would be right after the shower, just in case anything leaks in." We nodded diligently, but were still downright scared about having to deal with the catheter on our own. Little did I know, hygiene wouldn't be the problem. In fact, it wasn't the Hickman itself, at least not at that point; it was the tape.

In three days, as promised, we went back to the hospital, and the nurses removed the tape. It was so painful I almost screamed. The tape left a bright red circle about three inches in diameter around the insertion point of the catheter. It had completely irritated my skin, creating an acute allergic reaction. I won't describe it here; just imagine the skin of a burn victim. "Let's go through the cleaning procedure," one of the nurses said, beckoning Terry to come closer. A nurse applied alcohol to a cotton ball, and when she rubbed it over my raw skin, I nearly went into shock. The pain was so intense that I think my noseprint is still embedded in the ceiling of that exam room. My verbal reaction is not printable. Once I calmed down, one of the nurses said, "But this has to be sterilized; we can't let you get infected, even if it's painful." "But there *has* to be an alternative method. I can't stand another swabbing with the alcohol, and I will *not* allow you to put the tape back on me," I said. "That's the standard procedure, but let me bring in one or two people who are experts at dressings and bandages. Maybe they'll have some other ideas."

A nurse practitioner and another medical paraprofessional[2] came in, looked at my raw skin, winced, and poured out their sympathy, making me feel better, for it was clear from their expressions that I wasn't just being a wimp. "This is one of the worst cases of tape reaction I've seen," the para said. "Clearly, we can't put tape back on." "Well, if we dress it just with gauze and use paper tape, there will be a greater risk of infection," said the nurse. "Well, they'll just have to clean it twice as often," the para suggested. "Wait a minute," I said. "Twice as often with that alcohol? This doesn't sound like a pleasant solution!" "No, we'll ditch the alcohol, too. We have another chemical that works nearly as well but doesn't sting anything like alcohol." They left the room and came back a few minutes later with a long device that looked like a miniature version of one of those metal detectors people use at the beach in the hopes of finding lost coins and jewelry. They explained to Terry that she should remove the device from its packaging, squeeze its plastic handle, which would cause the nonalcoholic fluid in the handle to flow into the one-inch pad of cotton at the other end of the device, and then rub that over the skin around the catheter. The para did it the first time, and while I can't report that it was a walk in the park, the pain wasn't even remotely as bad as it had been with the alcohol a couple of hours earlier. "The skin needs air to heal," the para said, "so Terry, what you should do is put gauze all around it, secure the paper tape outside of the zone of irritation, and sterilize it frequently with these pads." Terry nodded.

I can't help but thinking now, several years later, that this was yet another more expensive solution I had painfully "earned": This cleaning device was obviously much more costly than a small alcohol pad in an aluminum packet that one can buy by the dozens for a dollar or two at a drugstore. However, in situations like this, I agree that one should begin by trying the cheapest products and making substitutions only if there is a need. Even if painful, the alcohol was not lethal, just a treatment from hell for someone like me with raw skin—and I did get the better product when it became clear that the cheaper alternative wouldn't work satisfactorily. So I do not oppose cost-effective procedures, at least not when the lowest-cost methods aren't jeopardizing a patient's health and costlier alternatives prove to be no more effective.

Although the fancy cleaning sticks were no fun, my red skin healed in about a week, and eventually each cleaning was no longer an exercise in self-control. Actually, the Hickman *did* prove to be a convenience. Given all the blood tests and chemical injections that needed to be done daily, it certainly was nice not having needles constantly stuck into my arms. After a week and a half, the Hickman was no longer my enemy, and Terry and I became pretty good at cleaning it. We got through that phase just in time to use the Hickman catheter for the first major part of the bone marrow transplant: the mobilization chemo.

Killing Me, One Chemo at a Time

Before my stem cell fluid was removed in apheresis, I would be getting the mobilization chemo, which was simply a megadose of Cytoxan—about ten times the amount I had gotten with each of my CHOP chemotherapies. By that time in my treatment, I already had pretty significant peripheral neuropathy—tingling in my fingers, pain in my feet, and the feeling that I was wearing socks even when I was barefoot. This is a typical side effect of the CHOP drugs, particularly vincristine. My peripheral neuropathy was so bad that when I walked the Dish trail those days with Paul, Anne, and Terry, after a mile or two, I felt like I was walking on coals, and I kept thinking my socks were bunched up under the soles of my feet when they were right in place. I could just imagine what it was going to be like during the mobilization chemo, when the 7,500-milligram dose of Cytoxan would essentially kill my marrow. (I would still have enough stem cells floating around in my blood to keep me alive, although there was still a chance that I could get dangerously sick from the temporary immunosuppression.)

Peripheral neuropathy was the least of my worries. After a few days of virtually zero infection-fighting capacity because of the mobilization chemo, the stem cells remaining in my blood would slowly begin to reingraft, but they would be starting from a much lower level than they did during my first six chemos. Because I would have virtually no immune system, I would have to stay at home and avoid people, especially anyone who was sick, as well as animals, dust, salad, and any food that contained live bacteria, including yogurt. Then, after about five days, when my few remaining stem cells started to find their way back into my marrow, I'd get double doses of Neupogen for five days straight, which would activate a massive stem cell multiplication process.

The mobilization chemo gave us one last shot at killing off my cancer cells, and the Neupogen treatment following it would increase the probability that my remaining stem cells would quickly produce fresh new stem cells. Once I had enough new stem cells, the apheresis could begin. It all made good sense.

I was again warned that the only downside of the Neupogen was that it would cause such intense multiplication and stimulation of my stem cells that when they tried to reingraft in my marrow, I might feel an agonizing pressure in my bones that could only be alleviated with strong pain medication. That turned out to be another dramatic understatement. After the mobilization chemo, which itself was rather uneventful, I started on the Neupogen, and after two or three days of double doses, my back hurt so badly that it was almost impossible to move, and I was given heavy doses of Vicodin, a narcotic painkiller, just to make it bearable. However, since I knew this time that the pain was a sign that my stem cells were growing back at a rapid rate, and that was exactly what I needed for apheresis—a large number of clean, fresh stem cells for a higher reingraft potential after the next round of chemo and radiation killed most of the fast-growing cells in my body—the pain was not only tolerable, but welcome. My white blood cell count was measured every day when we visited the hospital, and in my mind, I made an equation correlating the intensity of my bone pain to the growth rate of my white blood cell count. Of course, this would not do me any good, I mused, but it was at least a mental distraction.

A Date with Dracula

I went in the day before apheresis to meet the nurses who worked in the unit where my blood would be sucked out, processed, and pumped back in. I felt even more confident about the procedure once I had done so. The nurses had a good sense of humor; they had named the apheresis machines Dracula, Drano, Leech I, Leech II, and so forth. A person *does* have to have some humor when dealing with diseases of this sort day in and day out.

Since my stem cell fluid was going to be sent to the new Isolex 300i lab, where my stem cells would be purged, and there was a rumor that the machine damaged a lot of stem cells, the nurses told me they needed to get a very good yield of stem cells from me in apheresis to be sure that there would be enough undamaged stem cells for a successful reingraft later on. I asked how long they thought it would take to gather enough stem cells and whether I would have to go through apheresis more than once. One of the nurses said apheresis yields vary from patient to patient; some have great yields the first time, and some have to come back many, many times. I expressed my worry that the longer it took to harvest the stem cells, the more time would elapse between my last chemo and my bone marrow transplant, and if I had any residual cancer cells, they'd have a chance to start multiplying. "That may be," said the nurse, who was not prepared to debate cancer theory with me, "but we have to have enough stem cells." "So after the first day of apheresis, you'll measure my stem cell yield and tell me whether I need to come in for day two or three or four?" I asked, the sense of urgency evident in my voice. "Unfortunately, you're coming in on New Year's Eve, and there won't be a technician in to read your stem cell count, so we won't have the results until January 2. Just to be safe, we may call you back for a second apheresis before we've determined the yield of the first." It was my luck to be scheduled on a holiday, when there was a chance that I'd have to get an extra blood-sucking that I didn't need. Plus, it meant two days of waiting for results and all the anxiety associated with it.

We went to the hospital on New Year's Eve, Terry with her knitting, and me with my tubes. I can't remember whether I was apheresed by Drano or Leech I or Dracula, but the nurses were all very satisfied by the deep red color of my blood, which apparently indicates a high stem cell yield. After four hours of apheresing, they sent me home and said, "Have a Happy New Year!" They told me that my white counts were probably very high, thanks to the Neupogen, so there was no reason for me to worry about getting sick, and it would be okay to go to a New Year's Eve party. But they gave me the usual precautionary advice: Wear a mask just in case anybody there was carrying around any sort of flu bug, and avoid any appetizers in which guests had been "double dipping."

We spent New Year's at the Ehrlichs'. Nobody there was obviously sick, and I was able to relax and even drink a little wine, although Sandra had warned me to go slow because my liver was still detoxifying all the chemicals from the mobilization chemo. We waited until the day after New Year's to go back to the hospital. "What's my count?" I asked the nurse on duty eagerly. "Sorry, the technician didn't make it in today, so we'll just do another apheresis to make absolutely sure we have enough stem cells, just in case the first yield wasn't sufficient." "What kind of yield do you need?" I asked. "Oh, about 2 million stem cells per kilogram of body weight. Some patients do better than that and some do worse, and when it's worse, we have to keep doing apheresis until we reach that 2 million mark."

While we waited for apheresis number two, Terry and I visited the Isolex room and talked with the Ph.D. in charge. He said we were the first people to show any interest in it, and he was delighted to explain everything. The way the machine worked was really clever. As discussed in chapter 6, the monoclonal antibody in Rituxan creates a protein that attaches to the CD-20 receptor on B cells, causing the patient's immune system to see those cells as invaders and attack them, helping to get rid of the cancer but also killing good B cells. A similar technique was used in the Isolex 300i, which would remove my stem cells from the cell and fluid mixture extracted in apheresis. A protein was fashioned that attached to a receptor site on a stem cell. An iron particle was attached to this protein, so that when the protein docked with the stem cells, the stem cells could be attracted by a magnetic force. My cancer was in my B cells, which would be like floating impurities in the stem cell fluid, so I wanted to know how the stem cells could be separated from them. That's where the protein- and iron-enhanced stem cells came into play. The Isolex 300i had an electromagnet inside it that would attract the iron particles, and hence the stem cells, but would leave most of the B cells behind. The stem cell fluid would then be washed, reducing the impurities to about one part in 100,000. *But,* I kept thinking to myself, *with millions of cancer cells, reducing impurities to one part in 100,000 could still leave hundreds of malignant cells.*[3] However, thanks to Sandra's intervention, which contributed to Stanford's purchasing the Isolex machine, we would at least get the level of impurities down very low, and that certainly made us feel better, as it would reduce my chances of having residual disease later.

The last step performed by the Isolex was the addition of a chemical that would remove the protein and iron particles that attached to the stem cells. Then the stem cell fluid would be ready to be reinjected. The only snag was that nobody was sure how many stem cells would be damaged by the procedure of attaching the proteins to them, sucking the stem cells against the wall of the Isolex, washing them, detaching the proteins, and so forth—hence the need for a very high yield when my blood was removed during apheresis. I had no idea whether I was comparable to the mythical average patient when it came to my stem cell yield, and because the technician was off on New Year's Day and simply didn't show up the day after, I wasn't going to know for yet another day.

We went back to the apheresis room, and Terry finished knitting a sweater while one of the machines sucked out my blood, spun it in a centrifuge, and gave it back to me, minus the middle-weight components like stem cells. "I really think your stem cell counts will be okay," one of the nurses said. "So I may not see you back here?" I asked. She said, "Well, it all depends on whether we've got it up to 2 million cells per kilogram of your weight."

A few hours later, when I was back at home, I got a phone call from the nurse who performed the second apheresis. "Wow," she said, "I think you've set a record. You have 11.6 million stem cells per kilogram of body weight, and, to tell you the truth, we didn't have the slightest need for the second day of apheresis. However, with the new machine, the more cells we have, the merrier. If nothing else, we'll have a backup bag of stem cell fluid we can use in case anything goes wrong the first time." "Are they going to use the Isolex machine on both the regular stem cells and the backup bag?" I asked. "I don't know," she said. "You'll have to ask them." I thought it would be better to treat the extra bag with the Isolex right away, so that if I ever did have to use it, it wouldn't give me my cancer back. I still don't know whether that second bag of frozen cells has been run through the Isolex machine, let alone gotten the PCR test. In the low-probability event that I ever need that second bag, I will see to it that it does get PCR'ed before a drop goes back into me—but no need to worry about it now, since I don't think that is a likely prospect. But with mantle cell lymphoma, you never know.

9 | Zap It to Me: Staring into a Hiroshima-Dose of Radiation

AFTER THE GOOD NEWS about my super stem cell yield, I went to see Sandra. "What's next?" I asked. "Have fun for the next two weeks," she said, "because after that, the radiation will begin. We typically do it about two and a half weeks after the mobilization chemo, to give your body, and especially your liver, a chance to recover. Thirteen hundred rads of radiation will damage all the fast-growing cells in your body. That reminds me: you need to visit radiation therapy tomorrow so the technicians there can make some special lead plates for you that will cover your lungs and partially block the radiation. Your lungs will get only half the dose of radiation that the rest of your body will get, which reduces the chances of permanent lung damage." "But what about any cancer cells that might be hiding in the marrow of my ribs? If I'm going to have lead plates in front of my lungs, won't that reduce our chances of killing any cancer hiding in there?" "Yes, but there's a technique for dealing with that. Ask the radiologist."

Radiation Rehearsal

The next day, Terry and I went to Stanford's radiation therapy department and met with the radiology team members, who explained their techniques in detail and calmed many of my fears. As Sandra had explained, I was going to get thirteen doses of radiation stretched out over five days rather than having one huge dose all at once, which would reduce the likelihood of horribly severe side effects, although the radiologists didn't deny that they'd be pretty bad anyway. The radiation would be given in the form of full-body X-rays, and the technicians explained what Sandra had mentioned about the danger of nuking my lungs. To avoid that, they would make one-inch-thick lead plates in the exact shape of my lungs that would block out about half the X-ray radiation. Of course, I knew that the use of one-inch plates was formulated for—you guessed it—the mythical average patient, but I couldn't really think of any test that could be done to assess my resilience in this area, so I never questioned the one-inch specification.

The radiologists got to work right away, and I noticed that in addition to making the big, thick lead plates that looked like a T-bone steak that were going to hang in front of my lungs, they were making some negative plates that were exactly the opposite of the T-bone steak. These were lead squares with holes cut into them in the shape of my lungs. I was confused. "So why would you block my lungs with one plate, and then use another one that irradiates only my lungs?" I asked, knowing that the process couldn't be as counterproductive as it seemed. "Good question," said the radiation oncologist. "When we use the plates that expose your lungs, we're not going to use X-ray radiation. We're going to use different radiation particles that don't penetrate very far. They will get into your ribs to help clean out the marrow, but they won't get past them and into your lungs, because they don't have enough energy to do that." "So you're using electron beams when you expose my lungs and X-rays on the rest of my body?" I asked. Startled, he said, "Yes!"

I continued, "And this is no ordinary X-ray machine. It sounds like a scaled-down version of a cyclotron." "Why, yes," he said again. "We actually call the machine a linear accelerator, but it works much like a cyclotron." "So, let me guess: the cyclotron produces high-speed electrons, which then hit a photoelectric plate inside the machine, making the X-rays that will be curved around in my direction by a magnet and will be used to hit everything but my lungs. Then, later on, you'll remove the photoelectric plate and run beta radiation through the negative plates to clean my rib marrow." "Precisely," he said. I felt rather pleased that I could remember some physics from my studies at Columbia University in the early 1960s. I thought to myself, *I should tell this to Leon Lederman*, who was my physics professor nearly forty years earlier and was a friend now—I think he'd laugh that I remembered some of his lessons.

The radiologist showed me into the radiation room for a trial run. The room was empty except for the linear accelerator, a machine about the size of a sport utility vehicle. I looked at the machine and thought to myself, *I don't believe in exposing the general population to an extra rad of radiation, but here I am agreeing to be exposed to 1,300 of them!*

Some Risky Arithmetic

I wondered how risky it was to receive 1,300 rads over the course of a few days, which got me thinking about the risks of dying from other activities. Later I got on the Web and found very rough estimates of activities that could increase a person's chance of death in any given year by one in a million. These activities are:[1]

- Smoking 1.4 cigarettes (cancer, heart disease)
- Drinking 0.5 liters of wine (cirrhosis of the liver)
- Eating 100 charcoal-broiled steaks (cancer from benzopyrene)
- Eating 40 tablespoons of peanut butter (liver cancer from aflatoxin)

- Spending 2 days in New York City during severe air pollution (air pollution)
- Traveling 10 miles by bicycle (accident)
- Driving 40 miles in a car (accident)
- Flying 2,500 miles in a jet (accident)
- Canoeing for 6 minutes (drowning)
- Receiving 10 millirems (mrem) (or 1/100 of a rad)^2 of radiation (cancer)

Let's use the last entry of this table to put some perspective on the radiation risk. A chest X-ray delivers about 8 mrem, so it increases a person's chance of dying in a year by a little bit less than one in a million or so (leaving aside the possibility that what is learned from the X-ray may substantially reduce your odds of dying). The average amount of radiation we inescapably get from cosmic rays from space that impinge on the Earth is about 26 mrem per year at sea level, but in the thinner air of Denver and other high-altitude places, the radiation dose is about twice that, and in an airplane ride at 39,000 feet, it is about 0.5 mrem per hour. For a person like me who flies about 200 hours per year, that's an additional 100 mrem, which by itself increases my chances of death from cancer to one in 100,000. Since I've been doing about 200 hours of flying annually for the past thirty years, I've compounded my chances of dying from cancer from flying. Did that cause my lymphoma? It's impossible to know, of course. Maybe it was the air pollution from spending twenty-six years in the New York City area? A food additive? A pesticide? Despite the interesting statistics, we simply can't know what caused our diseases in most cases. However, it is instructive to compare the risks of medical treatments like radiation to the risks imposed by everyday activities.

I was going to get 1,300 rads of radiation, which is about 100,000 times more than the amount of radiation that would give me a one in a million chance of dying from cancer. That is broadly consistent to the 5 to 7 percent risk of contracting leukemia from radiation that Sandra mentioned. This is a huge risk relative to most activities (short of heavy smoking, which I don't do), but it must be weighed against the benefits—a potentially big reduction in my risk of losing remission from the mantle cell lymphoma. I figured that in my own case, I was more likely to die without radiation treatment (by losing remission) than with it, so as Sandra, Terry, and I decided in our decision analysis meeting, the benefits of radiation still trumped the costs—at least that seemed most reasonable at the time.

Better Stand Still!

Back in the radiation room, I learned that the lead plates, weighing maybe 25 pounds each, were too heavy to strap to my body, so they would be suspended from chains in front of me, and I would have to stand perfectly still behind the plates for eight or nine minutes while the linear accelerator zapped it to me. I asked, "But what if I *can't* stand completely still? Won't the radiation hit the edges of my lungs? These plates are almost exactly the size of my lungs, so if I move, won't I be zapped?" "There's a possibility of that," said the radiologist, "so you'll just have to stand really still after we put you in position; try your hardest not to stray from that spot." *Being statue-still for nine straight minutes is not going to be easy*, I thought, *especially not when I'll be staring down the business end of a lethal radiation machine and I'll be connected to tubes of fluids running to the Hickman catheter*. I understood how vigilant I'd have to be throughout the radiation treatment, and I was glad I had two weeks to prepare myself for it.

A Date with the Past

During those two weeks, I had a welcome distraction from the impending treatment. I was contacted out of the blue by the National Center for Atmospheric Research (NCAR), the lab in Boulder,

Colorado, where I worked for twenty years before coming to Stanford. NCAR had received a grant from the American Meteorological Society specifically for the purpose of chronicling the lives of key figures in the meteorology and climatology communities, and I had been fortunate enough to be tagged as one of the people NCAR was supposed to interview. I knew it couldn't have been an urgent project, because three times over the previous three years, my former Ph.D. advisee, Linda Mearns, who still works at NCAR, and I had tried to find time for the interview, but we never managed to cross paths long enough to do it. The first time, she got sick; the second time, she came to a meeting just as I was leaving; and the third time, when we were really going to do it, I had just learned about my cancer and had to leave the Energy Modeling Forum in Aspen early, to make my first appointment with Sandra, and Linda arrived after I'd departed. So my story about how I helped initiate the climate research work at NCAR had never been recorded.

I got a phone call from the NCAR historical archivist, who knew about my and Linda's failed attempts to connect for the interview. She apologized on behalf of NCAR and expressed an interest in doing the interview soon. The archivist asked me if I would mind if my old friend and colleague, Bob Chervin, came out to do the interview the following week. I knew the timing couldn't be a coincidence. "So you heard I'm going to have a bone marrow transplant?" I asked the archivist. Silence. "Well, yes, but we're not exactly worried. It's just . . ." I said, "Actually, it's very sensible. I do have a chance of dying from the procedure, so if you want anything out of my head, getting it now is probably pretty smart." She sounded enormously relieved.

A few days later, Bob appeared on my doorstep with half a dozen tapes and a tape recorder. I must say I was delighted in NCAR's choice for an interviewer. Bob and I had arrived at NCAR on the same day—September 1, 1972—and together we helped develop NCAR's climate research effort, which is still operating and producing valuable information to this day. We reminisced for two and a half days—which is, it turned out, nine and a half tapes—and it was great fun to reflect on the whole history of climate work done at NCAR and by the entire meteorological community. Bob left two days before my radiation treatment was set to begin, and when he turned the tapes in to NCAR, they said I broke the record—a tape and a half longer than anyone else. They transcribed the tapes almost immediately, but I haven't yet found the time to edit the 300-page dictation. Maybe next year—now that having a "next year" is a probable event.

You're Still Alive . . . So Do Something!

There were days during my cancer treatment when I felt like crawling into a hole and avoiding the world, and maybe that's what my right brain needed once in a while. At the same time, I know that staying active— eating out, staying in touch with friends and family, light hiking, and yes, even keeping a normal work schedule—drastically improved my cancer experience. I'd recommend to anyone that if, during your treatment, you are feeling good enough, get out and do something! You're not just a cancer patient but a human being, and you owe it to yourself to keep your body active and your mind engaged. Just don't overdo it. Let your advocate and your doctors help you figure out how to strike a healthy balance.

In the Line of Fire

The bone marrow folks really knew what they were doing. By having me come in for blood tests, consultations, and other appointments in the weeks before my radiation treatment and the bone marrow transplant, my visits to the unit, interactions with the nurses, blood draws, hydration bags, and so forth already felt routine. But still, when it was finally time for the radiation, I was pretty worried, especially given that radiation was an outpatient procedure. I was nervous about having to stand still for nine minutes three times a day in front of the death machine that was eventually going to give me life, but I was much more fearful about having to go home afterward. In my research on the Web I had read about the grueling side effects of radiation—skin burns, nausea, headaches, fatigue, collapsed immune system, and so on— and I wondered if my reactions were going to be better than age normal again or if this time I would fare worse than the mythical average patient, making it difficult to be an outpatient. I supposed that the only way to find out was to do it.

Terry and I headed into the bone marrow unit early, where I was given my schedule for the day of radiation and then asked to lie on a bed. I presumed I'd be taken to the radiation therapy department in a wheelchair, but apparently the docs thought I was perfectly capable of walking down there myself, despite the fact that they had already attached my Hickman catheter to a liter bag of saline solution, which was hanging on a rack with wheels. Terry helped me change into the new bathrobe she had just sewn for me, made of a wonderfully soft fleece that we had picked out together a couple of weeks earlier. Wearing my snazzy bathrobe, tubes emanating from my chest, I followed Terry into the elevator, pushing my rack of fluids and tubes that flowed into and out of the mechanical infusion pump that regulated the flow rate. We went down to radiation therapy and checked in, and almost immediately I was led to the radiation room, where I was told to stand up on the platform looking at the linear accelerator. I again reminded myself that the machine was going to help save my life, but it did still seem like an adversary at times.

For being so spare, the radiation room was actually somewhat pleasant, with wallpaper printed in fall-colored aspen leaves on all sides. I tried to pick a point on the wallpaper on which I could fix my gaze so that I didn't have to stare into the linear accelerator. Having gone through the rehearsal without radiation, I knew the drill: stand still, grip the handles on the sides of the frame holding the lung-protecting plates to make it easier to do so, and avoid swaying more than a half inch to either side to assure that the lead plates are protecting the lungs at all times. But we were done with trial runs; now came the moment of truth.

Terry and the technician left the room and went into the booth from which the linear accelerator was operated. I heard a few noises and saw a light come on in the machine, and I wondered if it was on. All of a sudden, I heard a whirring noise and felt a weird sensation come over my body. All the hairs on my arms, particularly in the places where my muscles were tense from holding the handles, raised as if somebody had rubbed a balloon over them or I had just pulled a mohair sweater off too quickly. It was very spooky. I knew that the static electricity effect was not from the radiation itself but from electrostatic fields created in the coils inside the machine, but it was nonetheless a reminder that this was no game.

I stood there for nine long minutes, focusing on one of my favorite scenes on the aspen wallpaper and talking to the X-rays: "Guys, I know you can't distinguish my good cells from my bad ones, and I forgive you for that, but I *do* expect you to root out every mantle cell in every corner of my body, from behind my eyeballs to my lungs to every other place." I had to laugh at myself a little bit as I underwent this semireligious experience, but I knew that I didn't just have a left brain and that bringing my right brain into the act was just as important for getting through this and for my long-term recovery. So I communed with the linear accelerator and welcomed these otherwise hostile and deadly rays. The hardest part of the treatment itself, other than the psychological irreconcilability of deadly rays nurturing life, was trying to stand still enough. I worried about exposing the corners of my lungs to extra doses of radiation that could cause such damage that later on, even if they wiped out my cancer, I might be the mythical patient who died from the cure.

The nine minutes finally passed, and the technician came in smiling, helped me down from the platform, and said, "Walk back up to the bone marrow unit and get some rest." Again, there was no wheelchair in sight. "What will I feel?" "Oh, maybe nothing, maybe some fatigue, maybe some nausea." I promised the technician I'd let someone know if I was feeling bad and told him I'd see him in another three hours. Upstairs we went. I felt perfectly normal, like nothing had happened—no flushing, no overheating, no fatigue. Just a little relief. I told Terry about my hair-raising experience in front of the linear accelerator, and we passed the time chatting. We went through that routine three times that first day, and then they sent me home. To my surprise, I felt perfectly normal that night.

The next day, Terry and I went in again. I repeated the previous day's procedure in the morning but had a surprise waiting for me in my afternoon radiation session. The technicians had put up the square plate with the lung cutouts rather than the lung steaks, attaching them to the end of the machine. This time, I wouldn't be standing up; instead, I would be sitting in a chair. It occurred to me that if I was going to be sitting in the middle of the room, the beta radiation wouldn't effectively penetrate my lungs, since the rays were less powerful and could only travel a short distance, but it turned out I wouldn't be sitting in the middle of the room but rather as close to the machine as possible, with my chest pressed right up against the lung plates so the radiation could hit them. "What will this feel like?" I asked them. "Nothing," they said. "It'll just do its thing." I sat there hugging the machine, with my chest pressed tightly against it to make certain that the beta radiation came through and hit all my ribs. The treatment lasted slightly less than nine minutes this time, and I got through it just fine.

Then it was back through the halls in my sporty new bathrobe, up to the recovery room to rest, although I didn't feel tired, and back down to radiation therapy again. For my last treatment on that second day, the technicians brought out a different square plate with lung holes, one that I had not seen before. "This one's for your back." So this time I had to put my back against the machine, and the high-energy electrons zapped through the holes in the lead to kill cancer in the marrow in the back of my ribs. I was impressed that Stanford had such an excellent radiation protocol; the radiologists were working every angle they could to try to kill as much cancer as possible without taking me down in the process.

Back upstairs, I was admonished by the nurses to relax, although I still didn't feel tired. "Can I at least sit at the terminal in the other room and do my e-mail?" I asked one of the nurses. "Are you nuts?" "Well, maybe, but why not let me try it? Is it going to harm me? I feel fine." "Well, you should be resting, but if you do e-mail for a few minutes, I guess it's okay." For the next three hours, I caught up on my e-mail until it was time to go down for the last treatment of the day, which turned out to be the normal stand-up treatment. Back home again, and back to radiation therapy again the next day.

The treatments became routine, and after a while I hardly noticed when my hair stood on end during the stand-up rounds, but I couldn't help but wonder when things were going to get ugly. How long was it going to take for the radiation to kill my fast-growing cells and create some of the horrible side effects like mucositis and the collapse of blood properties that killed so many people in Hiroshima and Nagasaki? The horrible deaths caused by radiation-induced loss of platelets—clotting agents without which people bled to death—were not absent from my mind. I knew, however, that by the time those effects started to manifest themselves, several days after the radiation treatments were completely finished, I'd be in the hospital and my Hickman catheter would be connected to whatever fluids I needed. I was confident that the docs were well prepared to deal with any and all side effects of radiation, and that had factored into my decision analysis when I agreed to radiation.

An Editorial Digression—
Nuclear War and Civil Defense

In going through intense medical treatments, there is much time to think. I am going to indulge in a mini editorial digression, since my experience with radiation treatment reminded me of a very difficult time when I worked on the nuclear winter problem in the mid-1980s. Nuclear winter is the name given to the likely climatic side effects of a nuclear war: The smoke from fires in cities hit in a major nuclear exchange would blot out the sky, causing winterlike conditions, at least for a few days, even in the middle of summer, which would be detrimental to agriculture (and therefore food production and consumption), not to mention all the other unimaginably horrible consequences of nuclear war.

I thought to myself, *How many bone marrow units are there in the United States?* I guessed thirty. *How many patient beds in each of these units?* I guessed another thirty. So that meant that in the United States, maybe 900 victims of nuclear war could be treated safely for acute radiation sickness of the kind that I was getting on purpose—presuming, of course, the hospitals weren't destroyed. I shook my head, thinking, *Yet there are absolute imbeciles out there who have claimed that civil defense measures could "protect" the population from radiation and its side effects. In the wake of a nuclear war, how could the millions that would be exposed to this kind of radiation possibly be saved? What a dangerous and cruel delusion of the propagandists for "winnable" nuclear war–fighting strategies.*

In the 1980s, Richard Perle—at the time, we referred to him, not so affectionately, as the "prince of darkness"—and other architects of the Reagan nuclear war–fighting strategy, seemed to act as if radioactive exposure of this kind would be an acceptable loss—just another civil defense matter. If there were only 900, or even 9,000 clean-room beds in the United States in which people suffering acute radiation illness could be treated, how were people in

Watts and in Harlem and in Chicago, and even in the rich districts like Beverly Hills and Scarsdale, going to get treatment? Who would give the blood they needed? Who would provide the electrical power to run the machines? There would be horrible death on a massive scale.

The delusion of civil defense for nuclear conflict flashed before me as I stood there being irradiated, thinking about how I was going to be kept alive, basically on life support, getting infusion after infusion of someone else's blood components, in a hospital clean room for three weeks while my body slowly recovered its capacity to sustain me. The thought of trying to perform those procedures in the streets of a nuclear-devastated city made me livid at the absolute, callous stupidity of those who asserted that civil defense could mitigate the horrors of a nuclear war. There's only one meaningful role governments can play on the issue of nuclear war: Prevent it at all costs. Anyhow, the treatment ended and so, too, did this kind of thinking.

Four and a Half Down, Four and a Half to Go!

Finally my radiation was done. It was a Friday in January 2002. I was told that I needed to come to the hospital the following Monday for the first of two myeloablative, or lethal, chemos—that is, chemos that would kill any fast-growing cells still in my marrow, just in case there were any left after the 1,300 rads of whole-body radiation. The first chemical I would be given was Cytoxan, the same chemical I had been given in all six CHOPs and in my mobilization chemo. I wasn't too worried about it, because I had tolerated it pretty well before. I would spend the night in the hospital after the first myeloablative chemo, and afterward I would be sent home for two days, at which point my immunities would essentially collapse from the combination of the radiation and the megadose of Cytoxan. Then I'd go back to the hospital, wearing a

HEPA filter mask, to get a megadose of another chemical, VP-16, also called etoposide, which would wipe my system out so completely that I would no longer be safe to go home or anywhere other than the clean room at the hospital. By that time, I would begin to feel the full effects of the radiation sickness.

When I came in for my Cytoxan, the man in the bed next to mine was getting the VP-16. He was two days ahead of me in the routine, and I started to feel a little jealous that he was farther along, until he kept me awake most of the night with his horrible, miserable, reactions to the VP-16. My heart went out to the poor soul, who spent more time throwing up in the bathroom than I did trying to sleep through it. It certainly did not increase my desire to come back two days later for the same treatment.

In the middle of the night, I asked the nurse on duty if everybody who got VP-16 had the same terrible reaction as my unfortunate roommate. "Some hardly notice it, but some react even more strongly than him. You just never know. Don't worry about it; we'll give you a very powerful sedative beforehand, and we have all kinds of drugs to make you feel better and to get you through it afterward if anything does happen and you're feeling awful." I felt only mildly reassured.

I was discharged the next morning, and Terry and I headed home, knowing it was the last time I'd be able to sleep in my own bed for about three weeks. I guess I *was* a little more tired than normal after the Cytoxan and the radiation, but I still didn't feel particularly bad. Terry had the cleaning of the Hickman catheter down to an art form, and that didn't hurt much any more, so the only negatives were my worries about how bad the VP-16 was going to be and when the side effects of the radiation would kick in, although they still seemed an abstraction since I felt fine, even a few days after my week of bombardment by the linear accelerator.

With trepidation, Terry and I packed up to go to the hospital. When we got there, we checked in for my VP-16 treatment. I was given an intravenous dose of Ativan, a drug that had already been prescribed for me to take in pill form for mild anxiety from time to time, and that I knew I could tolerate well. It was only a milligram, comparable to the dose I had taken before. Of course, I should have thought of the Benadryl experience, where one 25-milligram drip of it made me groggy for an entire day because the absorption rate was so much higher when it was administered intravenously. My reaction to the Ativan, I later found out, had Terry and the nurses very worried, because they couldn't wake me up. As far as I was concerned, it was the greatest thing that could have happened. I woke up to learn that I had already been given the VP-16, and I was thrilled because I had had essentially no side effects, which was quite a relief after watching my poor, retching roommate two days earlier.

Paul Ehrlich came to visit later that day, as he did every day for the next three weeks, and I made the joke that I'd "used up half of them." "Half of what?" Paul asked curiously. "My nine lives. I've had two and a half lethal doses of radiation, and two lethal chemos. That's four and a half out of my nine lives." He smiled wryly, making a mental note of my feisty comment for the e-mail chain on the play-by-play of my progress that I didn't then realize he was running.

CHAPTER

10 | Hospital Arrest

Squeaky Clean (Room)

After being given VP-16, I was admitted to a clean room. The clean room concept was one that I was well acquainted with after working as an engineer at Grumman (now Northrop Grumman) Aviation way back in 1966. In order to keep dust and other contaminants from getting into spacecrafts' delicate machinery, assembly was done in a room that had positive pressure and tremendously filtered air. Engineers, technicians, and other rocket scientists clad in masks, shoe covers, and special dust-free clothing entered and left the room through interlocking chambers designed to keep out unwanted particles. The number of air changes that occurred every hour in these clean rooms was staggeringly large, so if any stray dust did get in there, it would be removed quickly.

The clean room was essential for me because, at least for the first ten days in the hospital, I would be so severely immunocompromised that any bacteria, fungal spores, or viruses floating on dust particles that infiltrated my system could be life threatening. On top of the protection offered by the clean room, my Hickman catheter would be working overtime, giving me prophylactic antibiotics, antivirals, and, as I was to learn later, antifungals.

The clean room was entered from the hallway of the hospital, where a door led to a small room called the antechamber, which contained a sink and some scrubbing gear. On the other end of the antechamber was a door into my room. The room itself was spare, a pretty typical-looking hospital room containing only a bed and a chair. There was nary a speck of dust anywhere, thanks to the many air changes that took place each hour. There was a bathroom that could be accessed from inside the room, so there was no reason for me to leave the clean room and risk breathing in the microbe-laden dust that lurked outside.

While the setup really wasn't too bad, I was worried about getting a severe case of cabin fever. At least my room had a wonderful view of the hospital's inner courtyard, which not only had many flowers (in California, they can bloom in January) but also some trees that still had foliage that provided cover for a number of warblers and other birds. I was surprised that the birds inhabited such a small space, but I was glad for it. It was fun watching them, and it gave me something—birdwatching—to look forward to doing when I got out.

The nurses helped keep my mind active by putting a chart on the wall on which they listed my white blood cell count, my red blood cell count, and my platelet count every day after they'd drawn my blood through the ever-convenient Hickman catheter. All of my counts were essentially zero, and seeing them plotted on the chart on the wall reinforced what I already knew: I was dangerously immunocompromised. I was glad to be in the clean room.

I was allowed to have visitors, but before they came in, they were required to scrub their hands for three minutes in the antechamber, don a gown to cover their street clothes, and put on a mask. That all made sense, although I was surprised that they were allowed to keep on their street shirts, pants, and shoes. They weren't even required to wear booties over their shoes. I often nervously thought, *Aren't their shoes, clothing, and bodies carrying bacteria, viruses, and fungi into this room that could be let loose?* I tried not to think about it because I was very happy to have Terry, Paul, and other friends visit me. After a while, most everyone knew the drill, and those who didn't were intercepted by Terry, who explained what was necessary. I hadn't gotten sick, if that was any indication of whether the system worked, and I just hoped that only minimal amounts of contaminants were entering with my guests and that the air changes in the clean room could take care of any dust particles hosting microbial hitchhikers.

The Man Behind the Mask

One day I needed to have a chest X-ray, and the doctors didn't think I should leave the clean room and walk down the hospital corridor to the radiology department—after all, the hospital is where the worst germs are. So a portable X-ray machine was going to be rolled directly into my room, which seemed like a good solution. However, the machine was so big that the technician and the nurses helping him had to open the outer and inner doors of my room simultaneously to get the machine inside. I thought that defeated the purpose of bringing the X-ray machine in altogether, as I probably ended up being exposed to a lot of germs anyway.

The technician looked at me while this was happening and quickly said, "Put your mask on." I dutifully obeyed, strapping on the pink HEPA filter mask that I always kept within reach. As soon as the inner door closed and he started to set up the machine, he said, "Okay, you can take your mask off." Paul and Terry happened to be there at the time, and they looked at each other and then looked at me quizzically. My left brain swung into action. "Wait a minute," I said to the technician, my voice muffled by the mask. "How many times does the air change each minute in this room?" I recalled from my flirtation with rocket science, when I visited the clean room that housed Grumman Aviation's lunar excursion module—the vehicle that eventually took the astronauts to the moon—while it was being built. That room was incredibly sterile and underwent air changes every minute or so, and that was back in the 1960s, so I presumed the technology had advanced significantly. The technician didn't know a thing about the air changes—which could be expected, given that he specialized in X-rays and was probably untrained in the workings of clean rooms. About thirty seconds later, one of the medical residents walked in, so I asked, "How many air changes per minute do we have in here?" The doc wasn't sure, but he thought that a full change occurred about every five or ten minutes. I said, "So if both doors were open just a few minutes ago and some of the dust from the hall got in here, do you really think it's okay for me to take my mask off as soon as the second door is closed? Let's say a full air change happens every minute. Should I then take my mask off after the first minute?" "It's probably a good idea to leave it on a minute or two longer," the doc said. "Shouldn't I leave the mask on for ten to twenty minutes if the real objective is to make sure I don't get exposed to dust particles?" The doc furrowed his brow, and I was instantly reminded of some of my more trying discussions with some of the oncology Fellows. Rather than argue with him, I decided to cool it and dropped the subject, just hoping that my questions might get the hospital staff to thinking and eventually improving the routine for others.

Paul echoed my dust particle concerns: "They're not making us scrub our feet, they're not making us change our clothes, and they obviously don't understand how a real clean room functions." I agreed, and I could feel my irritation growing. "But," Paul reminded me, "be comforted by the fact that most of their procedures are helping to leverage the odds substantially in your favor. If you do what they tell you and, in addition, you leave your mask on for ten or fifteen minutes after any potential contamination, you'll improve your odds even more." "Precisely," I said, and this is in fact what I did for the remainder of my two and a half weeks there. I wore my mask for at least ten minutes after both doors were concurrently open and at least five minutes after the first door had been opened and the second one rapidly opened behind it. Overkill? Perhaps, but that was the only killing I intended to have happen in that room.

Once a nurse asked me to explain my extended period of mask wearing to her, and when I told her my logic, she said, "Seems reasonable to me. Why haven't the doctors made that the rule?" "I don't know; you ought to ask them. I tried, and I got a shrug."

A Dose of Common Sense

Sometimes common sense may be the best medicine. Your doctors *do* want what's best for you, but as you might have guessed by now, you can't assume that their systems are flawless. If something doesn't make sense to you or your advocate, ask about it. If there's something (e.g., extended mask wearing) that makes you feel more comfortable, ask your doctor if it's okay (i.e., not detrimental to your health), and if you get the thumbs up, do it! You may be tilting the odds slightly more in your favor.

I've often thought of life as a roulette wheel containing a bunch of wonderful opportunities mixed with some pretty terrible risks. Of course, we all hope that when we spin the wheel, the ball will come to rest on the good slots more often than on the threatening ones. Although nothing we do can fully eliminate the nasty slots, in cancer—and climate protection, for that matter—we can make the good slots wider and the risky ones narrower by learning about the issues involved and acting to improve the odds of better outcomes and reduce the likelihood of bad ones. There's no way to guarantee only positive outcomes, because sometimes terrible situations are inevitable, but the more we can slot the roulette wheel of life in our favor, the better.

—|—

When I began my stay in the clean room, I was handed off to the E1 wing of the hospital, meaning I was out of the day care bone marrow unit, out of the oncology unit, and entirely under the aegis of the twenty-four-hour bone marrow wing. There was a whole different set of docs, mostly young, whom I enjoyed enormously, but I knew they were neophytes and had little time to study Bayesian updating or concern themselves with residual particles remaining in the clean room even after a "complete" air exchange. I also became increasingly fond of the nurses in E1, both for their caring and their good sense. They dutifully plotted my white blood cell counts, which stayed close to zero for nearly a week; administered the prophylactic antibiotics; and explained upcoming procedures.

In fact, I had only one negative experience related to a nurse during the entire period I was in the hospital. It happened around the third day I was in the clean room, and thankfully, my left brain sensed there was a problem. I knew about every pill I was taking and could identify each one by sight, because when the nurses gave me my first cupful of them, I asked what they all were and why I needed them. On day three in E1, one of the better nurses, who was handling the ward with one nurse missing, came in with my usual cup of pills. Everything looked normal at first glance, but before I swallowed them I noticed an unfamiliar red one in the mix. "What's that?" I asked. She said, "Well, those are the pills that were prescribed." I said, "I've never had a large red pill before. Something's wrong." She didn't argue with me but rather told me she appreciated that I was paying attention and that she'd check it out immediately.

About ten minutes later, the nurse came back, red in the face and with tears in her eyes, and said, "Oh my God. I can't believe it. This isn't common, but it does happen. I accidentally switched one pill; the red one is meant for the patient in the room next to yours." I asked, "Well, how do you go about filling these cups?" "Normally, there are two of us, and we line up all these little pill containers and manually insert the pills, but we're short-staffed today, so I did it alone." "It's very easy for anyone to make an error like that," I sympathized. She said, "I don't even know what's in that red pill, or whether it would have been harmful to you or not, or whether the person who really needed it would've been harmed by not getting it, so I'm sure glad you caught it."

I had no intention of reporting the nurse for one minor slipup—she had been nothing but wonderful to me time and again. Besides, any human institution is going to make human mistakes. What bothered me was the method for filling the pill cups—simply lining them all up and dropping pills in manually. That struck me as an error-prone procedure, even if done by the most meticulous of nurses, and an example of a medical procedure that could be revisited by an operations research industrial engineer or some other qualified management professional. Coming up with more foolproof systems using information technology would sure beat having patients suffer unnecessarily or having nurses break down in tears thinking that they almost destroyed a patient because of their own error, which, in reality, is a flaw in the standard operating procedures they are forced to follow.

According to the Institute of Medicine, somewhere between 44,000 and 98,000 Americans die in hospitals every year as a result of medical errors, and medication errors alone account for about 7,000 of those. The National Committee for Quality Assurance, an independent watchdog group, estimates that in 2003 the failure to deliver best-practice care resulted in the death of 57,000 Americans. Until better systems are devised to reduce these fatal mistakes, patients and their advocates must continue to be vigilant at all times. Write down or memorize your medications and check before you take anything. Not often, but occasionally, you might just catch a life-threatening, albeit inadvertent, human error.

A Practical Solution to an Impractical Problem

One day, one of the nurses mentioned that I should be connected to a morphine drip. "Morphine?" I recoiled in horror. "That'll wreck my powers of concentration." I was still spending three hours a day on the phone and two hours doing e-mail, and my two assistants came to visit for half an hour every other day to help keep me caught up. "If I'm on morphine, how am I going to get my work done?" Over the next few days, other nurses also suggested morphine, but I still said "no way." "You're making a big mistake," one nurse said. "Just wait until the mucositis has fully kicked in." "I'm beginning to feel it," I admitted. "Do your gums hurt yet?" I confessed that my gums were getting raw and achy, but I still didn't know what the big fuss was about.

I'd been instructed from day one in the clean room to cleanse my mouth with a "lolly," a pink foam cylinder with ridges that was attached to what looked like a lollipop stick. I was instructed to soak the lolly in a special salt-water solution and to spin it around all the corners of my mouth and on and under my tongue in order to keep everything clean. "Why not use a toothbrush?" I asked. The nurses laughed in my face. "Just wait for your mucositis to kick in; then you'll understand," they said lovingly. So, three times a day, I went over to the sink, dragging my rack of bottles and tubes with me, and lollied my mouth.

I was very careful walking to the sink—and doing much of anything, really—with my arsenal of medical equipment attached to me, as I was paranoid about having an accident with the Hickman catheter after a conversation with one of the nurses. "Be careful not to step on any of your tubes," she warned me. "You don't want to pull your Hickman catheter out before it's time." "Ooh." A shudder went down my spine. "You mean I could pull it out?" "Yes, you certainly could. That's how we take them out. We simply yank them out when patients don't need them any more." A double shudder went down my spine. "You mean it's not surgically removed?" "Nope, the docs just pull them out," she confirmed. I commented on how painful that sounded, but she reassured me that removal wasn't too bad: "Just a sharp pain and then it's done." Now I had something new to worry about, or two somethings, rather: yanking my Hickman out prematurely and having it yanked out later, when we were through using it. There was also a third worry I had forgotten about: a contaminated tube.

By the third day in the clean room, the Hickman catheter was no longer my main worry, as I was getting full-on mucositis, and the lolly was really starting to hurt. My whole mouth felt weird, and it was excruciatingly painful to spin the torture lolly around in the corners of it. Soon the experience became even less pleasant. Bits and pieces of the inside of my mouth started coming off during the spinning, and I began to understand why radiation sickness was such a horrible way to die. My throat became so sore that I could no longer swallow without analgesics. The nurse again asked, "Can we connect you to the morphine? Please?" "I don't need it," I said. "It's just painful, not unbearable. I can get through this without it. I can't stop working." The nurses obviously put in my record that I didn't want morphine, because one of the young docs on duty came in and said, "If I was worried about getting mucositis, I would start taking morphine *before* I had any symptoms," trying to tell me I was being an idiot. Terry was pleased that the doctor brought it up, because she had been trying to get me to take the painkillers as well. But I was writing a very long and detailed rebuttal to the polemical and misleading writings of the Danish statistician Bjorn Lomborg[1] that was going to be part of a group effort, to be published in *Scientific American*, exposing his errors and misrepresentations. I couldn't allow my brain to dull. It helped my recovery to feel needed out there in the real world.

One night I tried to get to sleep once Terry had left after her usual fourteen-hour stint at the hospital. The mucositis had progressed to the point that swallowing was agonizingly painful; it felt like someone had turned on a drill in my throat that exacerbated the rash lining its walls. I didn't want to call a nurse and admit that I needed a painkiller after rejecting it for so long, so I was very glad when Janet, the senior nurse with whom I got on famously, came in on her usual round. I said, "You know, I'm beginning to think better of this morphine moratorium." She said, "Can't sleep? Can't

swallow? Can't drink? Can't eat?" "Yes." "Let me see your mouth."
I opened my mouth, and she shined her flashlight in and said,
"Hamburger." It made me laugh, which hurt. "You ready for morphine?" "I guess so, but can we make a deal?" "What's that?" Janet
asked. "Well, I'll need the morphine to sleep, but I don't ever feel
that bad during the day after I've been up for a while, so I
shouldn't need much in the middle of the day." She said, "How
about this: I'll set you up for a low dose during the day and a high
dose at night. When you really feel bad, you can just push the button connected to the morphine drip. It will give you up to three
extra doses in an hour." It was a perfect compromise and an indication that the senior nurse was willing to take a Bayesian approach. I wished the early negotiations with some of the docs had
been that easy, flexible, and reasonable.

Within ten minutes, the morphine pump was brought in, and
shortly thereafter, the Christmas-tree-like rack of wires and tubes
connected to one or the other of my Hickman catheter pigtails
now included a morphine drip. The nurse set it for a medium dose.
I didn't feel anything different. She said, "It takes a little while.
You'll notice it eventually."

The next thing I "noticed" was that it was 6:00 a.m. and I had actually slept through the night, thanks to the morphine. A different
nurse came in and asked how I was doing, and I told her about the
previous night's decision. "Glad you finally got smart," she said.
"You are one of the smartest people I've ever met, but I didn't
think your decision about morphine was very sensible. I understand
you want it low during the day, so I'm going to set it lower now, but
if the pain gets bad, let me know." She slowed the morphine drip,
and even with the reduced dose, my pain was quite tolerable. Indeed, my mouth hurt more with the lower dose, and indeed, the
mucositis was taking its toll on everything from the bottom of my
gut to the top of my mouth, but it was bearable. I could still log on
to e-mail, joke with Terry, Paul, and others when they came to visit,
and take care of about two hours of phone calls a day. I'd just press

the morphine button when the pain became unbearable. It was a pretty good solution to a bad situation—most of the time.

Just Say Yes

In the hospital, the street rules about "just saying no" to drugs don't apply. Sometimes more drugs can *improve* the quality of your life, especially if you are able to find a solution that allows you to be coherent when you want or need to be. Once your pain is out of control, it can be very hard to bring it back under control, so don't feel like you're a junkie when you just say yes. Your body and mind will thank you.

Fungal Fits

Around the time my mucositis started getting bad, a few of the young docs came in with a vial and reinjected my cleansed stem cell fluid back into me. That was the extent of the bone marrow transplant (autologous stem cell rescue). After all the preparation leading up to it, the procedure was done in a matter of minutes, with very little fanfare. The docs told me it would take eight to ten days for my stem cells to reingraft, and until then I was in substantial danger of infection, having zero immunities—hence the precautions with the mask and the prophylactic antibiotics and antivirals. I thanked them, not sure how to feel; the bone marrow transplant was definitely an anticlimactic event.

Life in the clean room went on for a couple days as normal, with everyone's attention focused on keeping me from getting any sort of infection or experiencing severe pain. One evening, right after Terry and I watched a tape of *Northern Exposure*—Terry had been dutifully recording reruns for me at home, which we watched together as a tremendous diversion from reality when my morphine was too high for me to work anyway—a nurse came in with an antifungal medicine for me. She explained that my immunocompromised state meant there was a risk I would contract a fungal infection in my lungs. I asked if any of my blood tests had indicated that I was developing an infection. The nurse said they hadn't, but they didn't want to take any foolish risks. I didn't argue. "Okay, do whatever you need," I said. "I just want to let you know that some people have reactions to this medicine," she warned. "Reactions?" I quivered, thinking back to my first experience with Rituxan. "Yeah, you just let us know if you have any tingling, shaking, chills, or other weird feelings." Since I'd tolerated the chemos after the first one and most of the other medicines very well, I presumed this was a standard warning, like the ones found on the inserts included with all medicines, describing all the horrible possible side effects, even though they're so uncommon that they're not worth much worry.

The antifungal was fed into my Hickman catheter, and about every half hour, the vigilant nurse returned to make sure I was feeling okay. After about two and a half hours, when there was only an hour or so left of the drip, the nurse came in and asked, "Still nothing?" I said, "Nothing. Is this like Rituxan, where people get vomiting reactions?" She said, "Well, yeah, it can be." "Well, the Rituxan hit me right away. I've had this for two and a half hours already, so I'm sure I'll be fine," I surmised. "Well, the truth is that patients often experience bad side effects about three hours into the drip, so just watch it. Call me immediately if anything changes." "Okay." We went back to watching *Northern Exposure*, and sure enough, ten minutes later, I started feeling shaky. I was glad that Terry had decided to stay later than usual. "What is it?" she asked. I said, "I don't know. I feel weird, shaky." Within a minute, I was shivering uncontrollably and my teeth began to chatter violently. I was horribly frightened because I thought that my tongue—already "hamburger" because of its disintegration from the radiation—was now in severe danger of being bitten off. Terry jumped up to get a nurse, but before she made it out of the room, I said, "Afraid . . . bite . . . tongue." Terry looked around the room and spotted a plastic bag containing a tube that was supposed to be used for emergency intubations of patients who had serious pulmonary flooding. She ripped the bag open and gave me the tube, and I put it between my teeth. My teeth were still chattering hard against the plastic, but at least I knew I wasn't going to bite off my tongue.

At some point during this episode, Terry had pressed my nurse-call button, and seconds after she gave me the plastic tube to chew on, a nurse came in and said, "That's what we were afraid of." She gave me an injection of a strong analgesic, Demerol, and it helped, but it wasn't enough. Terry asked the nurse if she had a dental device that would be better for me to chew on. She did, but not on my floor. "Can you order one?" "Give me a minute." She walked out the door, walked back in almost immediately and said, "I ordered one. The in-house pharmacy's open, and they're going to bring it up." Less than ten minutes later, a hard, wedge-shaped piece of rubber about five inches long and half an inch thick came. I put it in my mouth, letting my teeth chatter all over it, without the pain of jamming down on the hard plastic tube that Terry had found, though I was thankful for her improvisation, which saved me from eating the "hamburger" that was my tongue.

I was given another Demerol shot, which made me so groggy I could hardly move, and about half an hour later, the symptoms disappeared. "How often does this reaction to the antifungal occur?" I asked the nurse, bleary-eyed, sometime after 1:30 a.m. She said, "Well, it happens with at least half the patients." "Half!? Isn't there an alternative drug that could do the job?" "Well, actually, there is, and we're going to give that to you tomorrow and the next day, because you need three days of antifungal medication." "Well, why didn't I get that drug in the first place?" I asked. "I don't make the rules; I just carry out the protocol set by the doctors." I said, "Let me guess: I had to 'earn' it because it's much more expensive." "Bingo. It's at least three or four times more expensive." "So I went through this and almost bit my tongue off to save the hospital another 300 bucks?" She said, "Take that up with the docs; we just do what they tell us." "You bet." I took that up with the docs, big-time, the next day.

Around 2:00 a.m., when I was so drowsy that I was almost unconscious from the Demerol, Terry picked up the phone and called home, waking up her brother, Bryan, who was visiting for a few days, both to support Terry and me and to deal with his Silicon Valley business enterprises. Earlier in the day, Terry had promised Bryan that if she was still at the hospital after 2:00 a.m., she would call him and he would come sit with me and let Terry go home and get some much-needed rest. Bryan arrived around 2:30 a.m., and he stayed with me through the wee hours of the morning, agreeing with Terry that if I was unconscious, something was wrong and I needed to be watched. Bryan sat, keeping an eye on me while he caught up on some paperwork, and Terry went home and managed to get six hours of shut-eye.

One of the most important things about cancer treatment and recovery is support and love, and the kind I was getting from Terry, Bryan, the nurses, Paul, and many other friends was really important. My kids, too, tried to be as supportive as possible. In the early stages of my cancer, my son Adam called and said, "Dad, what can I do to help? If you need me to come home from Oregon, I'll just take the semester off." I said, "No, no, Adam. What I'd really like you to do, and I think at twenty years old now you can, is to not need me for a while. Know that I love you and am thinking of you. If you can fend for yourself so that I can concentrate on getting through this, it would be the greatest gift you could give me." These sounded like harsh words coming from a father, but I knew he understood. Indeed, he called almost every day just to find out how I was. Adam came through in spades, as did his sister Becca.

(Another) Cost Confrontation

I made it through the night, and, as promised, confronted the docs about the antifungal medicine the next day. "I understand that this hospital has to worry about costs," I told the team of young doctors who came to visit me twice a day. "I know you don't make the cost-benefit decisions around here, but doesn't the hospital tell you that it makes decisions on the kind of drugs patients get based on some cost-benefit logic?" "Yes, it does." I said, "Do you believe that logic is fair and reasonable?" "It's hard to say, but the rules are the rules." "Do you know that there's a more expensive antifungal that typically does not cause the side effects I suffered last night?" I asked. "Yes, we do, and we administer it to people who need it." I said, "But 50 percent of people need it; you just don't know who they are in advance, and they have to go through what I did beforehand. I could've bitten my tongue off! Is that cost-beneficial, or is that just protecting the private costs of this institution once again without any regard to total value?" They were silent.

I approached the subject from a different angle to illustrate my point. "So, why don't we do this if the hospital is so worried about money: Why don't we have two protocols, A and B, that have equal chances of success. The only difference is that patients under protocol A will be given all the low-end drugs and will suffer all the nasty side effects like hives and bite-your-tongue-off episodes. They won't be given Neupogen, so they'll most likely have to stay home and miss work for a week after every chemo, truly degrading the quality of their lives, not to mention costing their employers thousands of dollars. Then protocol B will be for those people who want to kick in, say, $10,000 of their own money to make sure they get the more efficient and less side-effect-ridden drugs. They'll get the Neupogen, will feel more like human beings, and will be able to work. And maybe there should even be protocol C, for those who can really kick in a hefty chunk of money for the best possible drugs and smoothest treatment." "Well, it may not be fair to give the better chemicals only to people who can afford them." I replied, "Exactly, so why not just give them to everybody? Given that the cost of these drugs is minor compared to the cost of a bone marrow transplant, I can't see any cost-benefit logic in not administering them in the first place. Is it worth it to save a nickel here and a dime there at the expense of patients' well-being?"

The young doctors nearly ran from the room—they'd come to talk about my mucositis, not about the philosophy of their institution's guidelines for decision analysis, cost-benefit analysis, and treatment of social costs. When I cooled down some, it became clear to me that complaining to young doctors wasn't the way to deal with the problem. I believe this issue has to be publicized nationally, on television, and addressed to hospital administrators, HMOs, and Congress, preferably by senior doctors who understand the issues, could present the information coherently, and could really help change the system. At a minimum, Congress must stop protecting HMOs and medical establishments from being legally challenged for demonstrably bad practices, for that gives them free rein to worry only about private costs, when in fact any economist worth his saline solution knows that it is the sum of private and social costs that determines efficiency and leads to optimal spending scenarios.

Many would argue that rejiggering hospitals' current cost-benefit models would lead to higher spending on health care, which is unthinkable for many governments and populations. The U.S. Department of Health and Human Services reported that in 2003, health care spending rose by 7.7 percent over the previous year, to $1.7 trillion, or about $5,670 per capita. (About $515.9 billion of that was spent on hospital care, up 6.5 percent from the previous year.) That sum, $1.7 trillion, represents about 15 percent of U.S. GDP. While I agree that these numbers seem staggering, I believe that if some of the procedures I advocate were put into practice, costs would rise only in the *short term*. To prevent costs from rising to exorbitant levels, stopgap measures could be put in place. For example, health insurance companies could establish a cost-effectiveness ratio to guide treatment decisions. Any treatment equal to or less than a threshold ratio value would be covered, while any above it would not. Ideally, the health insurance industry would consider personal *and* social costs in determining the ratio and cutoff value. It is my hope that such measures would encourage more effective, individualized care, while at the same time preventing patient and insurance company spending from skyrocketing.

If my treatment cost $1 billion, there is no way we could have done it; such a sum could help treat thousands of AIDS victims in a developing nation or feed thousands in a drought- and poverty-stricken area. But if my treatment costs climbed from $300,000 to $305,000 or $310,000, a mere 2 to 3 percent, as a result of individualizations, and my personal life improved and my ability to work increased, would it be worth it? I would give a resounding yes!

Over time, controlled spending on individualization of treatments, better (if sometimes more costly) medicines, and other health care improvements would likely reduce long-term costs, if they shortened hospital stays and prevented expensive treatments from needing to be repeated, or at least delayed them.[2] In addition, keeping people alive and productive is itself a boost to the economy if we consider social, and not just private, costs and benefits. From this view, the argument for individualization of treatments and other protocol upgrades is quite robust: Why wouldn't any industry spend slightly more if it were likely to recoup its costs, and why wouldn't governments push for practices that would bring social benefits as well as long-term savings? This won't just happen on its own; it will take courageous legislators and doctors to go public and pass laws mandating it.

I am no expert in medical cost-benefit analysis or health care legislation, and my suggestions are based mainly on my observations from my experiences in the trenches. I offer them here in the hopes that medical and public health specialists will seriously consider them. That is one objective of this book—to further stimulate this debate (which I know is already raging in medical institutions around the world), not to provide answers to it.

11 | My Re-Birthday

Blood Feud

About five days after the reinjection of my purged stem cells (the autologous stem cell transplant), the nurses began giving me Neupogen. "What's it for this time?" I asked. "To stimulate your stem cells to reingraft," a nurse told me. "Is it like mobilization chemo? In another few days, will I start getting all this bone pain, which is a sign that my cells are growing back, and then a couple of days later, will I actually overshoot my white count?" "Well, everybody's different. It usually takes a little longer than that, like nine or ten days, but maybe it'll happen sooner for you." "Thanks," I said, appreciating the nurse's optimism.

I was given Neupogen twice a day. The day after my first Neupogen shots, my white counts were still zero. My platelets were so low that I had to get a bag of what looked like squashed cantaloupe fed into me through the Hickman catheter. The orangy fluid was actually full of platelets, without which my blood would not clot, and I could bleed to death just from bumping my head. Every time my platelet count got too low, I was given a platelet transfusion. When my red blood cell count got so low that I was going to have trouble getting enough oxygen to my brain, I was given a red blood cell infusion. On some days, I got both. All in all, I got about a half dozen bags each of platelets and red blood cells.

When the entourage of young docs arrived on the seventh day after the Neupogen shots had begun, I asked them about my stem cell reingraft, and they said, "Oh, it'll probably take ten days for your stem cells to fully reingraft, and then you'll need Neupogen for another three days after that." "But my back is already starting to hurt," I told them. "I think my white blood cells are already multiplying pretty rapidly." "It's too soon," they said. "It'll be several more days." Soon, the back pain was as severe as it had been after my mobilization chemotherapy, when the pain increased with my white count from day to day. I remembered my mental mathematical model—what is called a regression model—in which I had correlated my rate of white cell growth per day with my level of back pain. Although this was done purely for amusement at the time, I couldn't help but remember it, because now I was really starting to hurt. "What are my white counts?" I asked the nurse when she came in. "I'll take the test and see," she said gently. An hour and a half later, she rushed in and said, "Wonderful! They're not zero any more. They're around 50." I conjectured that, given my level of back pain, they'd reach 300 the following day and well over 2,000 the day after that. The nurse smiled and said she hoped I was right, although that wasn't the usual pattern white blood cell counts followed. We'd just have to take the blood tests and see. I asked to talk to the doctors about my theory, because I didn't want to be given Neupogen and be forced to go through the excruciating pain of stem cell multiplication if I didn't need it, and the nurse promised she'd let them know.

Later on, the entourage of doctors arrived, and I explained the pain/white-cell regression equation I had mentally created after my mobilization chemo experience. Smiles lit across all their faces—though I could see only the smiling eyes, as their mouths and noses were under masks—for what they saw was an ignorant patient sitting there and telling them that he had a homespun rule for predicting his white count on the basis of how much his back and hipbones hurt. They good-humoredly told me that I wouldn't be out of the danger zone for at least two more days and that I needed the heavy-duty Neupogen shots. I said, "But I can't sleep, it's so painful, and I'm telling you, I'm going to be up there tomorrow, way above the dangerous level, and then in the thousands the day after that." "You just can't predict what's going to happen," one of them said. I said, "Well, how about just one Neupogen shot per day, and if my counts don't continue to increase, then I'll go back up to two?" They looked at me like I was crazy, using some old grandmother's remedy in the face of their training and medicine-by-the-numbers science. Of course, my model was based on the experience of the one person I knew—me. I was pretty confident that I knew how to correlate how I felt with what my white count was, because I'd been through it before, meaning I now had two sets of data—past and present. It sounded like the perfect situation for Bayesian updating, if only the docs would fly with it!

I explained my theory to the nurses, who thought it sounded plausible. "Can we make a deal?" I asked one of the nurses. "Don't give me the second Neupogen shot in the middle of the afternoon when you're supposed to, because then I'll suffer for the next six or eight hours with this intense bone pain. Can you stall it until about 10:00 at night, right when the morphine is pumped way up, so that I'll be able to sleep through the pain?" It was a temporary fix, because I figured I wasn't going to need the Neupogen after the next day, when I was sure my count would be over 300. The nurse said, "Okay, that's a fair deal. We'll still be giving you the Neupogen, which is what really matters, and in reality, the docs never told us precisely what time it was supposed to be done." So I was granted my wish and wasn't given the second shot until just before I went to bed, when my morphine drip rate increased, and I slept through the night.

Reborn?

The next morning, a nurse came in and took my blood. An hour or so later, Terry arrived and went through her five minutes of scrubbing. By that time, she had taken to cleaning her shoes with a sterilized wipe; she thought that was a smart idea whether it was required or not. Shortly thereafter, the nurse came in with another nurse, and they excitedly ran over to the chart with my numbers on it and put down the number 250. "You were right!" she said. "You are at 250. You have reingrafted. Happy re-birthday to you!" They sang "Happy Re-Birthday" to me, and I said, "Re-birthday? My birthday's not for another three weeks." They said, "Yes, but when your stem cells grow back, we call it your re-birthday. It means the transplant worked and that everything is going quite well." It was wonderful. I had tears in my eyes and was so grateful for the kindness and compassion of the nurses and other support staff.

"You know," one of them said, "we heard about the Neupogen argument you had with the docs, and we thought you were absolutely right. They're nice but young, and they don't always listen to us. They just do what they're trained to do, and that's all. You listen to us, which is something we can't always get them to do." "Well," I said, "they're pretty young, but they do mean well, and they're smart and well trained. They just haven't yet learned that experience is often as important, if not more so, than what you just learned in school last month." (Of course, having good data is the best possible scenario, but that is rare for many different medical questions.) That integration of training with experience will come with time, and I hope it will make them good decision analysts. "Thankfully, there are people like you around who truly are patient advocates," I said.

A Silver Lining in the Cancer Cloud?

When Paul came in, he learned of my re-birthday, and later on, so did all the other people on Paul's e-mail list, and I started getting phone calls and e-mails and notes from them and others. I was hearing from people I hadn't talked to in decades, and they were saying things I might not have heard in the course of ordinary life. A few people wrote that they saw me on Johnny Carson's *Tonight Show* in 1977 and as a result were inspired to get into environmental science and have pursued it as a career ever since. People I didn't know told me how reading some of my books had made all the difference in the world because it changed their career paths, their philosophies, and their outlooks. They wanted to thank me and wish me the best of luck in recovering.

In the midst of all this happiness, I just started to cry. I felt like I had been at my own funeral and just walked out the door. If ever there was a silver lining in the cancer cloud, this was it: finding out from people how I'd influenced their lives, something I never really understood or accepted; I was just doing my job—one foot in front of the other in an endless climb. The outpouring of deep feeling and support from friends, colleagues, and acquaintances made me say to Terry, "You know, I'm beginning to think I'm going to get through this, but if I don't, I know my life was worthwhile. The thing that's so amazing is that I had no idea about any of this. I give speeches, teach my classes, do my thing, and don't get much feedback—except scorn from certain rivals—but now I see I have made a difference. To get all this thanks and encouragement is just fantastic."

A Left Brain Vacation

Just as the elation over my re-birthday peaked, the doc entourage reappeared. Of course, I couldn't help giving them a friendly little "I-told-you-so" about my white blood cell count, but they did not change their opinion. "Well, it may be 250 today, but it'll probably go back down tomorrow before it finally catches and goes back up for good," one said. "Oh no," I said, "my bone pain is way up there about five hours after the Neupogen. My white blood cell count will be in the thousands tomorrow, so could you *please* stop giving

me the Neupogen now, or at least cut back to one shot today?"
"Oh, no, you must have both; they're very important."

The nurse in the room smiled and winked at me. Of course, I got my second daily shot at 10:00 that night, not at 4:00 p.m. like I was supposed to, and the next day my count was 3,300. When I saw the 3,300 on the wall and the nurses congratulated me that day, the second day after my re-birthday, I thought my reaction would be delight, but it wasn't. Tears again came to my eyes, and I could not control my feelings. I was sad, I was angry, and I didn't know what was happening to me emotionally.

Terry suggested I call my psychiatrist friend, and I took her advice. I called Gary Wynbrandt, the same psychiatrist who had earlier given me good advice about how to deal with prednisone withdrawal. "Hi, Gary, I have very good news. My reingraft has taken, and I'm doing great." "I always knew you were a fighter and you'd get through this," he said, clearly overjoyed. I said, "I'm supposed to be ecstatic about this, but my feelings are a jumble. I'm glad I'm on the road to recovery, but I can't help feeling sad all the time. In fact, it's hard for me not to spend half the day crying, which is very uncharacteristic for me." "Look, Steve, the average person with cancer throws himself at the mercy of his doctors, his God, or at least just feels overwhelmingly sorry for himself. Most people don't let their left brains take over and manage their treatment or spend their time researching their disease on the Web, following every detail of their treatment process, suggesting changes to protocols, and doing mental models of their reingraft. They also don't have a biologist wife who spends hours a day on the Web—catching all the latest reports on their disease so that they can review them together and discuss what to present to their doctors and how. You haven't let yourself *feel* your disease yet. Finally, you're at a point where your body knows there's nothing more your mind can do. Just let it happen. Let the emotion flow. Let the anger and the hurt and the 'How could this happen to me?' come out now. It should've six months ago, but you didn't let it because you were working overtime to make sure you were properly taken care of. There's nothing you have to do now, so just let it happen," he repeated. "Okay, Gary, I'll try." "No, you have to promise me that when you get these sad or depressive or angry feelings, you will not think about work, you will not banish them from your head, you will not divert yourself, but you'll just let them come over you. If it takes a month of crying, it takes a month. You've got a lot of mourning to do." Four years later, I can attest that the mourning isn't over yet.

When the nurses, and especially the doctors, came into my clean room, I still put on a happy face, and I still continued to work, entertain my visitors, advise students, and answer e-mails on a pretty regular basis. But for about half the day, particularly when I was using the torture lolly to clean my incredibly sore mouth, watching bits and pieces of my insides slough off as I spun it around, I felt that I had a right to my emotional hurt, and I let myself cry. I realized that dealing with mantle cell lymphoma was more than an experience and a challenge; it was a life-defining, and even death-defining, event that had intense emotional repercussions that I simply had to accept. That I waited until I was temporarily "safe" to let my right brain react was probably a good thing.

But even during this period of grieving, the reprieve for my left brain didn't last very long.

12 | How Much Risk Is Too Much?

The Dangers of Recovery

When I looked at my progress chart once during the day, when my morphine drip was low and my awareness high, I noticed that my platelets were climbing from the 9,000 or 10,000 per cubic centimeter level, which required transfusions, to 30,000 and 35,000 (normal is 150,000 to 400,000), and I started to mentally extrapolate when I was going to cross 50,000. I tried to recall why 50,000 was an important number, and then I remembered Michael Jacobs, my internist, telling me that as long as my platelet counts were below 50,000, there was little risk of my blood clotting. I was no longer taking an aspirin a day, which was all I'd done in the past to prevent any clots from forming as a result of my sporadic atrial fibrillations.[1] This worried me, because I had noticed that when the nurses came to take my pulse, it was mostly an atrial fibrillation. I routinely put my thumb on my neck and felt my pulse, and I knew the nurses must have had a hard time counting it, because it was hard to detect the ventricular contraction, which pushes blood out of the heart and is the main component of what the nurses would count as a "heartbeat." The danger was that if my atria fluttered for long enough, clots could form in my heart, and when my heart returned to its normal lub-dub rhythm, it could actually push the clots out, causing a stroke. Before the transplant, I had afibs intermittently, but they never lasted more than minutes to hours, so there was never enough time for the formation of clots that could cause a stroke. But now the afibs seemed to be constant, my platelets were climbing, and I wasn't taking aspirin or any other anticoagulant, all of which, I reasoned, put me at risk.

Michael Jacobs had put me on an aspirin a day rather than prescribing Coumadin, an anticoagulant drug (originally developed to be a rat poison), because my atrial fibrillations weren't too bad, and my heart was otherwise normal. But what now? Unfortunately, Mike was on sabbatical on the other side of the country, and I couldn't really ask him for his advice on whether an anticoagulant was wise if my afibs were constant and my platelet numbers were growing.

When an intern came in to check on me that day, I mentioned that my platelet count was around 35,000 or 40,000 per cubic centimeter, and at that rate, it was going to be over 50,000 in another two days. I reported that I was also having atrial fibs all the time. The intern, who had done a cardiology rotation, listened to my heart and said, "Yes, you are in atrial fib." He went to check my charts, and when he returned he said, "Well, every time the nurses have taken your pulse, you've been in atrial fib." I said, "Well, then, don't I need to be on an anticoagulant?" "Atrial fibs are a pretty common side effect of bone marrow transplants. All of your electrolyte and chemical balances are out of whack right now, but they and your heartbeat will probably go back to normal in a couple of months, six at the most, so I don't think we ought to worry about it."

I looked at him incredulously and said, "Wait a minute. This is serious! My platelets are going over 50,000 in the next two days." "You don't know that; it could take longer." I said, "Yes, or it could be tomorrow. I have full afibs, and I could have a clot, and soon I will have enough platelets that the clot might be big enough that it could be thrown from my heart and cause a stroke when my heart returns to its normal rhythm. I didn't go through all this hell to die of a stroke that could've been prevented with an anticoagulant." The intern repeated that an anticoagulant wasn't necessary, as my atrial fibs were likely only a short-term side effect of my treatment. He told me again not to worry, as there was a very low probability of my having a stroke.

I asked the intern what, in his eyes, constituted a "low probability," and he said, "Well, the probability that you'd get a stroke from afibs is probably 5 percent or less." My left brain almost exploded out of the side of my head. "What's the probability that I'll be run over by a truck?"[2] I raged. He looked at me oddly, never having thought of such a thing. "Well, what do you think it is?" I prodded. "What's the probability of my dying in general, even in my condition?" "Well, I don't know," he responded, dumbfounded. "How about one in 1,000, one in 10,000, somewhere in that neighborhood," I answered for him. "Five percent? If there were a 5 percent chance that there was salmonella in your chicken tonight, would you eat it?" "Well, of course not." "Right. And what does it take to fix my 5 percent risk of a stroke? A common pill like Coumadin that's relatively inexpensive and has very few side effects if taken correctly!" "I see your point," he mumbled.

I asked to see Dr. L. Bing Liem, the cardiologist I had seen before my transplant. Dr. Liem had told me then that he was considering putting me on Coumadin when I had only partial afibs. The intern gave in. "Well, if you insist, I'll check with Dr. Liem and see what he thinks." "Thank you for listening," I replied.

Common Sense Says: Prevent Preventable Problems

A nurse came into my room about three hours later to tell me that I had an appointment in another hour with Dr. Liem. When the time came, I put on my mask, though I didn't need it as critically since my white count was over 3,000, and the nurse wheeled me over to Dr. Liem's office. I explained my dilemma to him, emphasizing that in another day, my platelet count would likely be over 50,000, and frankly, I was worried. My fears were not unfounded. "You should've been on Coumadin two days ago!" Dr. Liem said, clearly concerned. I said, "That's what I tried to tell the intern this morning, and he seemed unconcerned about a 5 percent risk of stroke." "Why would you want to take an unnecessary 5 percent risk?" he asked, alarmed. I agreed but figured there would be trade-offs associated with the Coumadin, so I asked about the side effects. Dr. Liem replied, "Well, relative to a 5 percent risk of stroke? Nothing. We'll just monitor you." I was pleased to see some sensible cost-benefit analysis at work in the hospital.

I headed back down to the clean room, feeling perhaps a bit too smug, but also frightened to think what might have happened if I hadn't intervened. I wasn't ready for yet another brush with death. I also thought that this was one of many examples during my cancer experiences of the need for integrated medical care. I felt that each set of doctors I saw—the cardiologists, the oncologists, the internal medicine specialists, and later, many others— acted as separate entities; nobody knew my complete medical history. I'm sure that most medical institutions give cost-benefit reasons for insufficient integration, but I imagine more effective coordination of care would result in better treatment for all patients. In my case, Terry and I performed this coordination function for me. You or an advocate can do the same. (For assistance in aggregating your medical information, see http://www.ihealthrecord. org, explained in the Guide to Web References at the end of this book.) I have been told that some institutions are working to improve integration across specialists, and I hope that responsible medical administrators are strongly encouraging this movement.

—|⊢—

The intern returned shortly after Dr. Liem departed. He'd been told that Dr. Liem recommended Coumadin, and he conceded that he had been thinking about our conversation and now agreed with Dr. Liem's and my logic, especially given my history. He explained how to take the pills, and that day, I went on Coumadin. The intern wasn't upset that he had been overruled by the senior doctor, and I honestly think he learned to be a better doctor that day. That is the whole point of having interns in teaching hospitals. I was pleased I could contribute to his education. I confess I felt a twinge of guilt about being so aggressive with this nice young man, but I think he and I could have both regretted it if I hadn't.

Actually, four years later, I am still on Coumadin, although a much lower dose, and my afibs are largely gone, though I do have them from time to time. It turns out that the latest medical research on anticlotting agents suggests that aspirin is not nearly as effective as a low dose of Coumadin for those who tolerate it well—and I tolerate it well, having no ulcers, bleeding, bruising, or other typical symptoms. It seems like a pretty good deal, given that it lowers my risk of a stroke dramatically with essentially no comparably risky side effects. That is a textbook example of proper medical cost-benefit analysis that Dr. Liem initiated and Michael Jacobs has sustained.

So even though Gary Wynbrandt had advised me to shut off my left brain for a while and allow my feelings to come out, my left brain couldn't stay down when it got wind of a potentially life-threatening situation. And honestly, my left-brain way of thinking conjured up some important ideas about the bigger picture. *Doctors need to apply decision analysis in their everyday practice,* I thought again to myself. *It is unfortunate that medical decision-analytic skills rarely make it from the theoretical level taught in some med school classrooms to the practical level desperately needed in doctors and administrators in all medical institutions.* The good news is that this situation is not so much an intellectual challenge as a cultural one. The idea of applying decision sciences to medicine is already well understood by many health professionals. However, it will take a major cultural shift to close the gap between theory and common practice. It is my belief that if the top doctors in the top hospitals insisted on better and more widespread use of decision sciences, the practice would quickly trickle down throughout the medical establishment.

13 | Can't I Stay Another Day?

BY THE SECOND WEEK after the bone marrow transplant, my mucositis was so bad that I couldn't even swallow water, let alone the cans of chocolate- and vanilla-flavored nutrient-rich fluid the nurses and Terry tried to feed me, so I had to go on TPN—total parenteral nutrition—which was a liquid containing proteins, vitamins, minerals, and other nutrients that was fed to me through the Hickman catheter. The fatty white fluid started pouring into my catheter, along with various prophylactic antibiotics, antivirals, and antifungals, and I began to wonder when I'd ever get out of my hospital arrest in this not-quite-sterile room at Stanford Hospital.

On the one hand, leaving was absolutely out of the question, for in addition to all the intravenous drugs and TPN, I still needed morphine to get through the night, and even a little bit to get through the day. My three to five daily trips to the sink to use the torture lolly on my mouth were still an ordeal, and the radiation had damaged my intestinal tract, so my bodily functions were so out of whack that I wondered if I would ever be able to be away from a bathroom for more than half an hour at a time. On the other hand, I have to admit that I began entertaining thoughts about when I could get back on an airplane. My white blood cell count was high, and I was no longer asked to use my mask when both doors to my room were open concurrently, although I did use it in the halls when I went out for daily walks with Terry. Emotionally, I was still overtaken for hours every day by my need to mourn, but I think that it was helping because I was beginning to accept what I'd gone through and how close I'd been to death. Having 40 percent of my marrow composed of cancer cells when I was diagnosed had finally registered—but not until after chemo, radiation, a bone marrow transplant, and what seemed to be a good recovery.

To help me cope with the boredom and the pain, Terry came up with a great project. We had ten years' worth of photographs, still packaged in their original envelopes, that had never been arranged in photo albums. Every day, Terry brought in a photo album and a year's worth of pictures, and we selected the best pictures and put them in the album, chronicling our life together since the early 1990s. It was an uplifting experience to recall all we had done and to think about how much more there was to do, and it reminded me how important it was to fight my disease, be sensible about treatments, get healthy, and get back to living. I was also motivated by my continuing contact with my kids, students, office staff, and other colleagues. I knew the global environment was still in a serious predicament, and I had more to say and do about it, but it was also my responsibility not to jeopardize my recovery by overdoing it on the work front.

"I'm Not Going Anywhere"

At that stage in my recovery, Dr. Karl Blume, one of the pioneers of bone marrow transplants at Stanford, was doing rounds in place of the Fellows. When he entered the room, I did a double take. "Dr. Blume," I said, "isn't this out of the ordinary for you, doing patient visits in the bone marrow ward?" "Professor

Schneider," he quickly retorted, "don't you keep up with the progress of your students, even after they leave school?" "Of course," I said, "I understand completely." "It's important for me to keep my ear to the ground, so I make the rounds every now and then to see what's going on. I try to visit all transplant patients who are nearing the end of their stay so that we can talk about life back in the real world." "End of their stay?" I repeated skeptically. "I'm not going anywhere when I can hardly swallow, I'm still on TPN, and I need morphine to sleep." "I didn't say *today*," he said with a kind smile, "but in a few days." "A few days? It'll be another week or two," I said, fear creeping into my voice. "No, I don't think so," he said. "You're recovering very well, and you're safe now that your white count is high, although we do still want you to be very careful, because not all the components of your immune system are back in order. It's time for you to start thinking about transitioning." I asked Dr. Blume what he meant by "transitioning," and he said that it was not just readapting to the real world but also accepting that I wouldn't be able to do all the things I used to take for granted. I would be very weak for a long time, and Dr. Blume guessed it would take my system anywhere from six to eighteen months to recover, so I'd have to configure my lifestyle accordingly.

Aha, I said to myself, *I think the nurses sent the heavy artillery in because they didn't trust that I would go home and rest, but would rather jump right back in the saddle as soon as I got there.* Dr. Blume continued, "You need to think of recovery over a long time horizon. What would take days to recover from with a normal disease will take weeks to months for you; the recovery period really is prolonged that much with bone marrow transplant patients. Some people never quite come back completely, although I think your remarkable response to the treatments and the strength of your body bode well for you and probably mean that you will fare better than most. But you still have to give it some time."

But When Can I Get on a Plane?

Then I asked the big question: "So when can I start flying again?" Dr. Blume laughed, teasing me for being afraid to leave the clean room yet talking about hopping on an airplane. I guessed that it would be another three months before I'd be safe to fly again, but Dr. Blume said three months was very early because bone marrow transplant patients sometimes have substantial problems with immune deficiency for many, many months after their procedures. There was no reason to take any unnecessary risk of getting an infection, he said, and I agreed, although I almost choked when he suggested that six months was a more realistic time frame. Dr. Blume explained that generally he advised people to stay home and not go back to work or get involved in any heavy activity or exercise for four months after their release from the clean room, and then slowly work back to their precancer activity levels.

"Four months!?!" I bellowed. "I have a class to teach in the spring quarter, which is five weeks away. There will be thirty-five students waiting to take my seminar, and I can't let them down!" "Can you let them give you a flu or a cold or something else that might threaten your life?" he fired back. "And do you really think you'll have the energy to prepare lectures, stand up in front of a class, and present your materials effectively?" I said, "I've done it here." He laughed again and said, "I heard from the nurses that you had seven visitors in here the other day and that everyone was talking and laughing at once." It was true: six colleagues who are also my friends happened to stop in on Terry and me at once, and I mused that the scrubbing room must have looked like Grand Central Station. I said, "You have a good spy network." He said, "You are notorious on this floor." "Yeah, but the company makes me feel good and picks up my spirits." He said the visitors were no problem but that I had to remember that my busiest day inside the clean room still couldn't begin to compare with a regular day outside of it.

I knew Dr. Blume was emphasizing the need to rest for a reason, so I tried to be agreeable. I promised I'd let my body be my guide, but I was going to try to teach my class and get back to my duties as a professor, and if I felt okay, I'd keep doing it. Dr. Blume wasn't thrilled with my answer, but he conceded, saying only that I had to throttle back if the teaching proved to be too much. I was less worried about the teaching than about my peripheral neuropathy; my hands were so weak that I couldn't open a jar, let alone play the twelve-string guitar, a favorite pastime of mine. Dr. Blume thought the peripheral neuropathy in my hands would improve with time, but we'd just have to wait and see about my feet. I figured we'd have to wait and see about a lot of things.

On his way out, Dr. Blume reiterated his warning: "The most important thing, Steve, is not to overdo it, because there's absolutely no way you're going to have your usual energy level. Your body has been devastated; we've kept you alive with IV drips, and you need time, and time alone, to heal. It'll take at least a year before you're feeling anywhere near normal." I deeply appreciated his flexibility, openness, and concern, and I understood why he was a well-loved and respected doctor.

I continued to tell myself that I was nowhere near ready to go home, despite Dr. Blume's thoughts to the contrary. After all, what was I supposed to do without the morphine and other drips feeding into my veins through the Hickman? But about two days later, somewhere in the middle of my third week in the clean room, which was a few days shy of what I was told would be my minimum stay, Dr. Blume returned. "Okay," he said, "*Now* I think you're ready to go home." I objected, pointing out that I was still connected to morphine, but he countered that I didn't need the morphine and they'd give me fentanyl and another, less strong painkiller anyway. He reminded me that I was able to drink some liquids and could probably eat baby food. *I guess I could eat baby food*, I thought, *but what about all my other symptoms? How am I going to deal with them at home? I'm able to get some fluids down, but not nearly enough to stay hydrated!* Dr. Blume must have been reading my mind, because he said they'd leave the Hickman in a while longer, and they'd send me home with a backpack with an electric pump that could be connected to saline solution. The saline solution could then be pumped into my catheter to keep me hydrated. I'd still come in to the ambulatory bone marrow unit every day to have my blood, fluid levels, and other vitals checked.

"You'll be all right. Just use your mask when you're going back and forth to the hospital, and be absolutely certain to wear it around your students. Oh, and make sure your dogs are nowhere near you at home." I continued to protest, wondering how Terry and I were going to adjust to this dramatically different lifestyle, even if it was temporary. Sensing my anxiety, Dr. Blume said, "Okay, tomorrow then. Not today, but tomorrow." I said, "But it's sooner than twenty-one days." "You're ready today, but we'll compromise. You leave tomorrow. Now, you have all night to think about it. Just sleep on it, and I bet by the time morning rolls around, you'll like the idea of getting out of here."

A Patient's Best Allies

That night, the nurses came in to say good-bye and to tell me that everything was going to be okay—and to warn me for the umpteenth time not to overdo it. I was touched when they told me how much they enjoyed interacting with me and hearing my often-true predictions about my body, and how appreciative they were of my willingness to listen to them, even when some of the docs wouldn't. I was saddened that not everyone treated them with respect, as it was the nurses—the primary caregivers, night watch people, sympathizers, and listeners—who were a cancer patient's best allies during treatment.

Reentry

The dreaded day of my departure arrived. Terry was there, as were several nurses and the exercise trainer. They had all come to say good-bye again and to wish me luck. I strapped on my mask, and the nurses made me sit in a wheelchair, which I thought was a joke, since Terry and I had been promenading all around the hospital for the past week in order to get some exercise and prevent muscle atrophy. But lowest-common-denominator rules are the rule, so I didn't argue. I sat in the chair, got wheeled out to the front, and was then set free from my not-quite-solitary confinement.

Terry started to drive home via our regular route, but I said, "Would you cut across campus?" She drove across the Stanford campus, and I saw students biking and playing ultimate Frisbee and other games, and it felt wonderful to be alive, but it also made me think about my cancer experience and wonder what might lie in store for these students or their parents over time. How many of them or their friends or relatives had already had the horror of experiencing what I went through—or worse? It made me realize how important it was to get on with my life and do whatever I could to help other people in similar situations increase their odds of survival.

—|—

I got home feeling pretty good, and went into the kitchen, where I tried to open a jar of baby food that Terry had bought for me to see if I'd be able to eat it. My efforts were futile. I didn't have the strength in my hands to open the vacuum-sealed baby food jar. In fact, I couldn't reopen the jar that Terry had already opened; the peripheral neuropathy in my hands was so bad that just twisting the cap was too much.

I found that I could write, but not very well and not for very long, but I *could* use the computer, because that did not require the squeezing ability that holding a pen did, just the finger-tapping on the keyboard. I logged on and tried to catch up on my e-mail, but it didn't last long. After half an hour I felt very chilled, so I put a blanket around myself, but then I got very hot and sweaty and had to remove it. I began to understand what Terry was going through with her hot flashes. My body's thermostat was completely out of whack, something Karl Blume had warned me about. *I wonder how long it'll take for that to return to normal*, I thought to myself.

The adrenaline from coming home wore off, and I had to ask Terry for help walking up the five steps to our bedroom and getting into bed. I took a nap, probably the first nap I'd taken at home in thirty years. I had to alternate between putting on blankets and removing them, trying to find the happy medium between shivering and sweating.

I awoke four hours later, astounded that I'd slept for so long, and realized that I truly was a lot weaker than I had thought. "We've got four weeks before the spring term starts," I said to Terry, "and I have to teach this class." "You're going to wait and see how you feel before you decide to do anything," she advised me. "I need to try to go for a walk," I said. "They said I need exercise." "Okay, but let's take it slow." We went outside that first day at home, and we started to walk toward the Stanford Dish trail, me with my mask on because there was dust blowing around, and Terry supporting me. I thought better of trying to climb the steep hill leading to Stanford's giant radio telescope, so I opted for the milder road that ran behind our house. Well, we'd gone about 100 yards from the house when we reached a little twenty-foot hill. I think I got ten feet up the hill before I nearly collapsed, and Terry almost had to carry me home. I needed another nap after that exhausting Olympic event. This one lasted about three hours. Being that weak was both debilitating and frightening.

Yet I got stronger by the day. The torture lolly still hurt like hell, the mucositis persisted, and my bowels were a wreck, but I was making progress. A half an hour sending and answering e-mails became forty minutes, which became an hour, which became two hours, and I even considered making an appearance in my office. The four-hour naps became two-hour naps. I started using a half-dose-strength fentanyl patch. When my frustration got the best of me, Terry reminded me of what Dr. Blume had said: "What you'd normally recover from in a day with most other diseases takes at least a week with this one. Have some patience." Unfortunately, patience had never been my strong suit.

Accept Your Condition, But Don't Settle for It

Indeed, I learned the value of patience in my first few weeks at home, when I felt the same as I always had mentally (aside from the mourning) but felt like I was living in the body of someone many decades older than I was. Not even all of Dr. Blume's warnings could have prepared me for the physical hardships involved in recovering from a dread disease and its grueling treatments.

Patients should take the warnings of their doctors about life after cancer treatment very seriously. While it will be necessary to take it easy, that is not a ticket to become a couch potato and stop trying! Just know your limits, and don't do anything so strenuous that you could jeopardize your health. Over time, if you're determined, you'll be able to push those limits more and more, and you'll feel your strength and energy returning, slowly but surely.

"One Good Hard Yank"

Every day, Terry and I went to the bone marrow unit, where I was given a blood test, and things were fine. But after a week at home, I started to feel flushed at night. The nurses had given me the thermometer that they'd used daily in the clean room to take my temperature, and I began to use it again. Normally, my temperature is one to two degrees Celsius below normal, but it began creeping upward—half a degree above normal, and then a degree above normal, which, for me, is in fever range. At that point, I was worried, so we went to the bone marrow unit early the next morning, and I told Karl Blume, who happened to be on duty again, about it. "I'm concerned about this," he said. "I'm going to take a large blood sample." My Hickman catheter was still in, so Dr. Blume used it for my blood draw, and I was sent home.

That night, my fever was quite spiky, and Terry was so worried that she suggested going to the ER. "ER?" I said. "You only go to an ER if otherwise you'll be dead. I can wait until tomorrow. I'm too exhausted to get out of bed right now." Early the next morning, we went to the bone marrow unit, where I checked in as an outpatient, and the friendly-but-scolding nurse who had dealt with me nearly every day in the clean room said, "The blood test that Dr. Blume took is back. It looks like you have a staph infection,[1] and he is almost certain it must be inside one of the catheter tubes. The catheter has to come out." I said, "But it's not scheduled to come out until next week." "Let me give you some advice: you don't want a staph infection with a direct connection to your heart." I wondered aloud how I'd get enough fluids without the catheter, and the nurse said we'd just go back to using IVs. Yuck. I tried a bit harder to dissuade her, because I remembered what they'd said about removing the Hickman: no surgery; it just gets yanked out. I had been so afraid of stepping on a tube and pulling it out, and now they were going to do essentially that!

One of the young Fellows, Alexandra Simic, whom we liked very much, was in that day, and she said she'd take out my Hickman catheter. I was glad it was her because I thought she was one of the gentler and smarter Fellows in the group. "So what do we do?" I asked once we'd gone into an exam room. "Just lie down, and I'll yank," she said. I reclined on the exam table and asked, "Now, what do I need to do?" She said, "Just don't think about it. I'll give one hard tug, and then it'll hurt a little at the insertion point, and that's it." She pulled left, right, center, harder, harder, harder. Ouch, ouch, ouch. Nothing happened. The nurses in the room said, "Sometimes it works if you really twist it around," and they demonstrated the twisting hand motion. The Fellow tried twisting my catheter around. Nothing happened. "Well, I'll give it one last tug," she said, exasperated, "and if it doesn't come out, we're going to have to send you to surgery and have it surgically removed, although I'm not sure giving you anesthesia is such a good idea, given everything you've been through." We all looked at each other nervously. The threat of the surgery completely overrode my fear of the pain of the catheter pull. "Oh, what the hell. Give it one good hard yank," I said. I shut my eyes and clamped my jaws shut, and the Fellow applied all her force to the tube. The Hickman flew out, hitting her in the face and splattering blood on her blouse. I felt bad, like we should pay for the dry cleaning. I was in a little pain, but not much, and I realized that my mind, as well as my nerves, controlled many of my experiences. The pain was nothing compared with the anticipation of it.

I waited for all my blood to come gushing out all over the bed, but nothing happened. The Fellow quickly put a gauze pad on top of the opening in my skin and applied some pressure to it, and after about five minutes, the wound was just slightly oozy. "Why isn't blood spurting out all over the place?" "That only happens in the movies," one of the nurses said. "The superior vena cava carries blood *into* the heart; if the Hickman was in the aorta, which pushes blood *out* of the heart, we would've had a mess, which is one of the reasons we put the Hickman catheter where we do." I was once again impressed by these very important nuances in medicine.

The removal of the catheter did the trick for my fevers. I had only one more night of fever, and by the next day, my temperature went back to normal. I was given a prophylactic antibiotic, just in case, and fortunately, the infection didn't wreak havoc on my weak immune system. Karl Blume's guess about the staph infection in the catheter was right, chalking up another point for the value of experience and understanding of process.

14 | Darth Vader in Pink

Hello, World!

Sooner or later, it had to happen. I couldn't spend my whole life at home, doing all my work over the phone and on e-mail, although I admit that not going into my office on campus and dealing with the administrative tedium that came with it actually allowed me to get more research and writing done and communicate more with students. However, the time had to come to terminate my spell as absentee professor and return to campus.

Later that week, there was going to be a seminar on campus, and I thought it was important for me to attend. I said to Terry, "Okay, this is it. I'm going to this one." "Are you sure you're up to it?" I thought I was as ready as I was ever going to be. The alternating hot flashes and chills were subsiding, I was able to "hike"—albeit slowly—for maybe 300 yards; I was certain I could make it in to the office and even take the stairs—well, maybe two flights max—if I had to, although the building does have elevators (which I used, of course).

On the day of the seminar, I headed out with my HEPA filter mask, which I had to wear for another three months or so, in place. I arrived at the seminar room a little early to apologize to the speaker for my appearance and explain to him that I had just gone through a hospital procedure and I needed the mask, but apparently somebody had already told him, and he didn't mind anyway. Later on, students and faculty filtered in, and when they saw me, they waved, and some even applauded. It was wonderful to see all those familiar faces again.

I listened to the talk with interest. At the end, there was an open discussion session, and after one or two other people had commented, I raised my hand. Several people looked over at me, including Paul, and they must have been thinking, *He's not really going to ask a question with his mask on, is he?* I figured the idea of wearing the mask was to avoid breathing in germs, but when I talked, I'd be breathing out, so it would be perfectly safe to take it off while speaking. When I was called on, I took a deep breath through the mask and then lifted it about a half inch off my face. I made a breath's worth of comments, replaced the mask, took another deep breath so quickly that nobody even noticed, finished my comments, asked a question, and replaced the mask. Everybody heard what I had to say, and my system worked just fine. When the seminar ended, I milled around and talked to people and concluded that my first outing was a success. I hoped that the dry run had prepared me for the real test, which would begin in three days, when my class started. *I can do this!* I said to myself, thinking Karl Blume would be pleased with me for carefully testing the waters, and for waiting three weeks before doing so.

After attending the talk, I was confident that I could spend a little more time on campus, so I started going to my office for a couple of hours every day, feeling good about just having a visible presence around there for the first time in many months. I was still strict with my visitors, warning them not even to *think* about setting foot inside my door if they were the slightest bit sick. I promised ailing students and colleagues that we could talk over the phone or e-mail or in person when they were over their illnesses. The fact that I was willing to see them at all a few weeks after the bone marrow transplant, when the doctors' advice was to stay home for a minimum of four months, meant that they had to go along with my request. Everybody was wonderful about it. Students got used to seeing me out and about with my mask on, and prospective graduate students tolerated the mask just fine when I interviewed them. I took the mask off only when I was absolutely sure that the person I was meeting with had no infections, and usually only if the meeting was in my office. Given that I stayed healthy, I'd say it worked out pretty well.

Debating About Precautions

Before the academic quarter started, I had another appointment with Sandra Horning. Now that I was out of the clean room, I went back to seeing her in the oncology department. She and Terry and I discussed the last couple of months of treatment and recovery, and she said she was thrilled with my progress but—as you might have guessed—that I shouldn't overexert myself. She repeated Dr. Blume's orders almost verbatim: If I insisted on teaching, I was to keep the pink mask on and stay away from dust and anyone with an infection.

Sandra also wanted me to come back in four weeks for a CT scan. Our long-running debate over PCR resurfaced at the mention of the CT scan. "But Sandra, the probability that the CT scan will reveal anything now is pretty low, unless the whole bone marrow transplant was a failure, right?" "Yes, it's very unlikely that it will show anything." "Why don't we do a PCR and find out if I have any cancer cells for sure?" I reminded her of the extra frozen cancer-infected lymph node sitting in Ron Levy's lab. I wanted that PCR'ed, as well as my supposedly cancer-free blood, so that we could compare them. I said, "I know you can do PCR if my colleagues in the biology department can do it." She gave her standard answer about not knowing exactly what the PCR results would tell us. "It means that if we start to see exponential growth in my cancer, we'll know that we should start doing maintenance therapy," I told her. "Oh, that again." We went around and around about maintenance therapy: about the lack of data and about whether it might trigger the untoward growth of non-CD-20 B cells—something Sandra and Ron Levy both thought was possible but exceedingly unlikely. I repeated my cost-benefit arguments and even suggested that given the relatively low toll Rituxan would take on my health, we should do it prophylactically, just in case I had any residual cancer. Sandra's answer was: "We don't treat people who aren't sick. Besides, we don't know that the Rituxan will work as maintenance therapy." I argued back that she didn't know that I wasn't sick, and unless we did a PCR, we'd never know until large lumps reappeared, which would require intensive and expensive treatments. In addition, I was willing to take a chance with Rituxan for maintenance therapy. Despite the lack of frequency data to prove it, I was convinced that the Rituxan had contributed to my excellent results up to that point. This was a replay of our previous conversations on the subject.

Terry and I still didn't get the problem solved to our liking, but at least we departed with Sandra promising that she'd think more about it. In the early days of our relationship, "I'll think more about it" meant that some, but not a lot, of thought was likely to go into my questions and suggestions. But after we had our excellent decision analysis discussion, when Sandra said she was going to think about something, I believe she really spent a lot of time pondering it, and her behavior—deviating from the standard protocol on a number of occasions—proved it.

School's In

Finally, the first day of the class I was coteaching with my friend and colleague Armin Rosencranz rolled around. I showed up wearing my pink mask and saw that about forty students were already crowded into the room. I told the students my situation and explained that I probably would not have many office hours but that they could e-mail me anytime, call me anytime, and visit me in my office provided they weren't carrying around any bugs. "In fact," I said, "if any of you are sick right now, with a cold, fever, or other bug, please leave the room. Don't worry about missing anything; I'll give you a private lesson later on what we cover." Two students gathered up their belongings and left. One of the sick students called later to go over the material, and the other said that he didn't need a review of what I'd discussed because he'd heard me give two lectures before, and he'd heard from the other students in the class that I'd covered much of the same material that day.

By and large, the first day went well. The students were unfazed by the mask and even seemed thrilled that I was willing to teach in my condition. One young woman came up to me after class and said, "Listen, Darth Vader in pink, your agreeing to do this for us speaks volumes. We really appreciate it." "You've got it backwards," I told her. "I can't be cut off from you guys. You represent the generation that's going to inherit the mess that my generation has made, and if you want to learn about that mess and how to fix it, it gives my life purpose, because that's what I want to discuss with you guys." Having these refreshing, honest, and intelligent young people back in my life was a huge boost.

I made it through that first two-hour lecture, but I was very glad Terry came to pick me up, because I wasn't sure I would have had the strength left to drive myself home. *Maybe I'm overdoing it*, I thought. Of course, I couldn't admit it to anyone else, because I already knew that most of my friends and family members thought I should be home resting, and I had every intention of proving them wrong. Since the class ran only from 6:00 to 8:00 p.m. on Tuesdays, I figured I could save up enough energy in the week preceding it to get through it. I added a Tuesday afternoon nap to my strategy, and that's how I handled the first weeks of the term: sleeping from 3:00 to 5:00 on Tuesday afternoons, getting to class at 6:00, lecturing for a couple of hours, and then going home and collapsing. Eventually, I was able to make it home and eat dinner after the Tuesday lectures before running out of steam.

Culture Clash

I went back to see Sandra again in mid-April 2002, and she said my progress was good. She thought that I was probably pushing a little too hard, but as long as I didn't get sick or overly exhausted, it was okay with her. She gave me the go-ahead to ditch the mask, even during class, although it would still be smart to wear it if there was any serious risk of infection, and certainly I should continue to wear it around construction sites, of which there were dozens at Stanford at any given time. Sandra also said I didn't have to worry about avoiding foods with bacteria in them any longer because my white count was more than high enough that I was not going to get sick from them. Little did Sandra know, I had made yogurt, which contains the bacteria *Lactobacillus acidophilus*, part of my diet long before then.

When I returned home after my time in the clean room, one of the stern warnings I was given was not to eat foods containing live bacteria—uncooked meats, fish, uncooked vegetables, salad, and even yogurt. But my bowels were a wreck, and in the past, when I had traveled out of the country and gotten Montezuma's revenge, which is just what this radiation-induced bowel disturbance felt like, I always found that eating a couple of yogurts when I came home solved the problem after a day or two, and I never needed medication.

About a week after I had come home from the clean room, I'd gone in for my daily appointment in the bone marrow unit and asked the doc on duty, "How about yogurt?" "Oh no, no live bacteria for a month." "But my system's a disaster. I can't be more than three minutes away from a bathroom without feeling like I could be at risk of an accident. This is not an acceptable way to live, and I think the yogurt will fix it." "No bacteria," the doc repeated.

Later I ran my idea by a smart and experienced nurse in the bone marrow unit. I thought that two spoonfuls of yogurt twice a day would probably be enough to help with my bowel problems. My white count was up around 2,000, and even though that was half of normal, it was well within the safe range, and I couldn't fathom how "friendly" bacteria could hurt me anyway. "What are they worried about?" I asked. "This whole notion of avoiding *all* bacteria is completely overblown. Shouldn't you be more specific about what bacteria to avoid?" The nurse thought I was absolutely right, but there was no way she was going to suggest violating the protocol, because it was like Scripture in the bone marrow unit.

Feeling thwarted once again, I had taken my case to the senior doctor on duty, a flip but brilliant Canadian and an esteemed bone marrow transplant specialist. I told him my theory about acidophilus aiding bowel recovery, fully expecting another "no" when I asked about the yogurt. "You know, I've always thought the bacteria rules for transplant patients were a bit overdone; there's no reason to include foods with acidophilus in them on the list of forbidden foods. Why don't you give the yogurt a try for a couple days and see what happens, and if it cures you, great! Your white count's not so bad that it could do any damage anyway." So that day I'd gone home and eaten two scoops of yogurt, and two more the next day. The day after that, while I couldn't say that things were back to normal, my poor gut was dramatically improved.

But back to my appointment at Sandra's office. Once again, we had a short discussion about maintenance therapy and PCR, but to no avail. "I don't think we can stall much longer," she said. "Stall about what?" I asked. "Your bone marrow biopsy." "Oh, I need another one of those?" I asked grimly, my back already beginning to ache. "It's exceedingly unlikely that it'll show anything," she said, "and frankly, I think we'll learn very little from a biopsy done only three months after your transplant, but that's what the protocol says, and you're signed up under this research protocol now, so we should probably follow through on it." I said, "You mean I can't be used in the database if I don't have the bone marrow biopsy?"

"Precisely." "Okay, fair enough. You've helped me out; this is the least I can do."

Terry and I headed back to the bone marrow ward, and not Oncology Day Care, for the bone marrow biopsy, because the research protocol I had signed onto for the Isolex was technically being carried out by the bone marrow unit. I took a deep breath and wondered how, just hours earlier, I could have been on cloud nine. The day before my appointment with Sandra, I'd received a phone call at 6:00 a.m. from my longtime friend and colleague Susan Solomon, the same Susan Solomon who led the expedition to Antarctica in the late 1980s that proved that the ozone hole was caused by manufactured chemicals like the chlorofluorocarbons (CFCs) used in refrigerators. "Steve?" She said. "Yeah?" I answered, confused, looking groggily at the clock. "I figured you wouldn't mind me waking you up to tell you that you've just been elected to the National Academy of Sciences." In science, that is about the highest possible honor awarded, so I was ecstatic. But the elation had all vanished by the next day when I realized in Sandra's office that I was going to get drilled in the back with a large-bore needle again. It brought me back down to Earth in a hurry and gave me perspective on the emoluments of professional recognition; while they were important and I did feel incredibly honored, their significance receded in the face of medical issues.

Before the bone marrow biopsy, the nurses in the bone marrow ward did something that was never done for me in the Oncology Day Care Center, where I had the other two bone marrow biopsies: They gave me a fentanyl "lolly." It was literally a lollipop, made of a hard, spherical lump of fentanyl-laced "candy" attached to a stick. I was to suck on the fentanyl until it completely dissolved in my mouth and all of it entered my system. I knew the lolly was going to be a good thing, because I had recently asked Gary Wynbrandt about it. "Gary, I'm going in for a bone marrow biopsy tomorrow, and I was wondering if it would be okay to take a couple of Ativan beforehand to calm me down." "Yeah, that could be helpful," he agreed. "It's not a painkiller, but it might make you a little bit less stressed." I said, "Well, they're going to give me a fentanyl lolly for the pain." He laughed out loud and said, "Well, if they're going to give you that, don't even worry about the Ativan. If fentanyl were a brick, Ativan would be like two flies landing on it." He told me fentanyl was an analgesic about eighty times stronger than morphine, so I knew I was going to be more comfortable during the bone marrow biopsy than I had been before, when I was only given Novocain and told, in essence, "Grin and bear it, kiddo."

It took about fifteen minutes for me to eat the lolly and feel its pain-quelling properties kick in, and then it was time for the drilling. This time I was told to lie on my side instead of on my stomach, and then I was given Novocain. I still can't say that the procedure didn't hurt like hell, but my pain level wasn't even in the same ballpark as it had been during earlier bone marrow biopsies. Removal of the aspirate was no fun, but I figured I could endure just about anything in life for fifteen seconds, and at least this time I wasn't dreading the results, as I was confident that my cancer count would be zero.

Too Little, Too Late?

About a week and a half later, I had my next appointment with Sandra. She congratulated me on my election to the National Academy, and then we got down to business. "We have the results of the bone marrow biopsy, and your cancer count is zero!" she exclaimed. "That's great, Sandra, but it's only zero according to the eye of the technician who . . ." She cut me off: "I think I've found a way to get PCR for you. You said Ron Levy has a piece of your lymph node?" "Yeah." She thought there was yet another research protocol for which I could sign up that would allow us to do PCR on the cancerous lymph node as well as on my blood, so that we could finally compare my pre- and posttreatment cancer cell counts. I was pleasantly surprised. "Thank you, Sandra. That's wonderful." She cautioned that it would take them a while to analyze the results, but she promised to get it done and let us know the results in another couple meetings. "It's still not clear what the PCR numbers indicate, so we'll have to feel our way through it." I of all people couldn't object to subjective analysis. "I'm very glad we're doing this," I told her, though I was thinking, *Why couldn't I—in fact all patients—have gotten PCR earlier so that we could have checked the stem cell fluid before it was reinjected during the transplant?*

15 | A Delicate Balance

Flying Days

I was feeling so confident about my recovery that the first question I asked Sandra the next time I saw her was, "So, when can I get on an airplane?" Sure enough, after the excellent bone marrow biopsy results and my white counts' movement up toward the low end of normal in May 2002, my flying days began again. Terry's and my first trip was to New York to see my dad, and I was slightly nervous about it. I never told him flat-out that I had cancer, but I did tell him that I underwent a hospital procedure that I termed a "blood cleansing." My dad also knew that the procedure had prevented me from flying on airplanes for three months. He accepted it all over the phone, but I was worried about what questions he might ask in person.

In addition to seeing my dad, I would be seeing my brother and his family and Sanite, the loving and responsible nurse who had been caring for my father for the past five years. Terry and I also had to meet with some editors from Oxford University Press, and I had a lecture to give somewhere too—just a typical multipurpose trip.

On the one hand, stepping on the airplane felt completely normal—so normal that I couldn't believe that I hadn't flown for eight months. On the other hand, every time I heard a sneeze or a cough, I became paranoid and reached for my mask, even though

I was no longer carrying it around. The long-term immunosuppression was not just physical; it had gotten into my psyche, and I worried about what might happen to my sinuses or my lungs on that plane ride. In truth, now, three years later, I still wince at sneezers in my vicinity.

Fortunately, the trip went very well, and I arrived at my dad's still feeling good. At the time, I hardly had any hair, and I was still wearing berets and baseball caps to cover up the reality of what my life had been like for the past eight or nine months. I figured my dad wouldn't notice it, because at ninety-four he wasn't as aware of things as he had been, but I was wrong. After a day or so of catching up with my dad and being told how glad he was that I was now able to visit again—and if he could only know how glad *I* was to be able to visit again!—he said, "Is something wrong with your hair?" "No," I stammered, "I just had a haircut that turned out to be too short, and as a result, I'm cold, so I like to wear a hat." "Oh, I see. That makes sense. So do I."

Itching for Relief

While I was thrilled to be traveling again, there was a significant negative aspect to the trip. It began with a bit of redness on the inside of my right wrist, which started to spread up my arm. My skin became really ugly, blotchy, and rough. And itchy. Very itchy. Soon, the rash appeared on my left arm, starting at the wrist and then moving up my arm, just as it had on the right side. It hurt, it was hideous, and it concerned me. I had gotten used to living with the "minor morbidities" of the bone marrow transplant, including atrial fibrillations, lowish white and red blood cell counts, peripheral neuropathy, a poor thermostat, significant edema (swelling) in my feet, ankles, and left wrist,[1] lack of energy, and the hair loss (although the hair was very slowly growing back). Severe allergic dermatitis had never been on the list of possible side effects, but there it was, and boy, was it annoying.

When I got home from New York, I immediately scheduled an appointment with my friend Dr. Joann Blessing-Moore, who specializes in treating allergies and asthma. Joann took one look at my rash and said, "Ew, you should get this biopsied. Let's make sure it's not shingles or something weird." I went to the dermatology unit, one of the outpatient clinics at Stanford Hospital, and got the rash biopsied, and two days later, just as the rash had become more painful and was beginning to spread to both my ankles and move up my legs, I got a call from the clinic notifying me that the rash was a severe allergic reaction. I phoned Joann and asked her what we should do, and she prescribed various antihistamines and ointments. I tried steroid ointments, nonsteroid creams, and three or four different oral antihistamines, but the rash just kept getting worse. Between the edema and the rash, my legs were noticeably swollen and absolutely revolting.

Joann continued to throw the pharmacological arsenal at the rash, but nothing happened. "Well, there's one way to control it for sure," she said, "but you won't want to do it." "What's that?" I asked, desperate for a solution. "Prednisone." "Oh, no, I don't want that stuff again," I said, "and it's probably not a good idea when my immune system is already compromised." So we agreed we'd use a massively aggressive treatment but wouldn't go for the whole-body steroid attack.

After a few days, the rash didn't seem to be getting any worse, but it was still pretty bad. I called the oncology unit to let Sandra know about it, and I got a call back from Sandra's Fellow. He said I had contact dermatitis and told me to change my deodorant and detergent and avoid using laundry softeners, including dryer sheets. Could it really be that simple? We dutifully rewashed all my clothing with a different brand of detergent and sans dryer sheets and followed all of the Fellow's directions, and it had about as much effect as the pharmacopoeia of antihistamines had: precious little. The rash got so painful that I scoured the drug stores until I found a Bactine preparation containing 2 percent lidocaine—a drug similar to Novocain—that I sprayed on my legs to reduce the itchiness and prevent myself from scratching so much that I'd be at risk of infection.

Finally, I had a chance to see Sandra in person about my rash. "Allergic hypersensitivity is not a standard bone marrow side effect," she said, "but we'll watch it." "There's a lot to see," I said, and I showed her the photographs we'd taken. "Oh dear," she said. "You may seriously have to consider prednisone." "I don't want prednisone," I said. "Well, if the rash becomes whole-body, you may have to." So far, it was still only on my arms and legs, but it *was* causing me quite a bit of grief.

On Fire

At the end of June 2002, when the rash was still wreaking havoc, Terry and I had to fly to a meeting in Boulder, Colorado, which just happened to be having its hottest summer and worst fire season ever. Of course, this was the perfect setting for a global warming meeting, and the irony wasn't lost on several of the participants.

The problem with the 100-degree weather and the fires in town, other than just being unpleasant, was that there was so much smoke in the air that I began having allergic reactions in my lungs. It started with broncospasms, of the kind I would normally only get after a severe flu, when I was no longer sick but my lungs were so irritated that they would produce secretions that made it hard for me to breathe for about a month after all other symptoms had vanished. It got worse and worse. I phoned Joann Blessing-Moore and told her I needed something to open up my lungs. She phoned in some prescriptions for lung sprays to a pharmacy in Boulder, but when I picked them up, I realized that the most effective one contained albuterol, a stimulant that would only make my arrhythmias worse, so I was unwilling to take it—especially on the road. I tried some mild steroid sprays and felt a slight improvement, but not much. It was hard for me to sleep, and if I was ever exposed to cold air at night or early in the morning, I would have a paroxysmal coughing episode.

I survived the trip—barely—and as soon as I returned, I headed to Joann's office, where I breathed into a tube attached to a spirometer—a machine that measures air flow into and out of the lungs—and discovered that my small airway passages were functioning at 70 percent of normal. Joann said that some drugs could bring my capacity back up to 90 percent, but that I'd still notice that I was below normal. "What could be causing this?" I asked. "Well, you've never had anything like this before, so the bone marrow transplant would be my first suspect," she said. "But the doctors and nurses in the bone marrow unit said this isn't usually a symptom of a transplant." "Well, nobody knows everything about the interrelatedness of bone marrow transplants and allergies," she replied. "By the looks of your skin, I'd say eosinophils are involved in the reaction." "What are they?" I asked. "Components of your blood that usually accumulate wherever allergic reactions, like those involved in asthma, take place." It turns out eosinophils are white blood cells whose natural role is to defend the body against parasites. (High levels of eosinophils can be a sign of parasitic infection.) During an asthmatic reaction, they can be released into different areas of the body, including the lungs, where they can cause serious problems. Her remark made me suspect that my changing white blood cell counts were causing imbalances in my histamines and eosinophils, although there was no way to be certain.

The Last Straw

I thought it was kind of like in climate theory: We know that the climate is a nonlinear system, meaning that sometimes one change doesn't do much, but another, similar one might push the system over a threshold and trigger a dramatic response. In other words, the stimulus and the response are not proportional. Our bodies are complex systems just like the climate, so I hypothesized that maybe my white blood cells, now climbing back to normal levels, had exceeded some threshold that caused my eosinophils and other allergy-related cells, including T cells, to go nuts. Joann suggested testing my "theory" by doing a series of blood tests, so every week for the next few months, I went in for a blood test. The tests showed that between June and August, my white count went from a below-normal level of about 3,000 up to 5,000 or 6,000. The allergies were at their worst up to that point in August, so my theory appeared to have some support.

My lungs got so bad that in September, when Terry and I were supposed to fly to a meeting in Illinois, I didn't think it was safe for me to be on an airplane. Terry and I both skipped the trip, and on the day we were supposed to depart, we went instead to see Sandra about my newfound lung problems. By that time, Sandra had gotten the results back from the PCR test that was done on my blood. "Phenomenal news!" She said. "Zero cancer cells!" That *was* phenomenal news, and I began to think, *Maybe I have beaten this disease*, but my itchy legs were a constant reminder that the aftereffects of my cancer and treatments still lingered. "Sandra, you told me that the marrow is scoured by Rituxan but that there still could be cells hiding somewhere. Maybe we didn't PCR enough fluid to find them." She didn't give me a chance to argue further. "Just be happy with these great results." She told me the lab ran the PCR on both the cancerous lymph node from my arm that had been kept by Ron Levy's lab and on my pretreatment bone marrow fluid, when 40 percent of my bone marrow cells were cancerous, and there were 800,000 cancer cells per microgram of DNA in the tumor and about 200,000 in the bone marrow fluid. But now, the PCR of my posttreatment blood revealed zero—actually, less than ten, which is considered indistinguishable from zero! "Come back for a blood test in another month, and we'll check again for cancer cells in your blood." She agreed that we'd continue to do the PCR tests, so if my cancer showed up again, we'd be able to detect it way ahead of the time a CT scan would.

After the PCR issue was settled, I asked Sandra about my allergic reactions. She said that my reactions were so bad that she thought the benefits of taking prednisone for a month would far outweigh the costs. At that point, it was seven months after my transplant, and I could not continue to live in misery with my rash, my edema, and my incapacity to breathe normally, so I gave in and agreed to the prednisone. I let Joann know that Sandra had given me the go-ahead, and she prescribed the prednisone for me. "Let's start with a high dose and taper it down," she suggested, and that's what I did.

The results were absolutely amazing. Within two days after starting the prednisone, *all* my reactions had ceased: no more broncospasms, no more horrible rashes, no more scratching. The prednisone was literally a miracle drug, but I knew that it was bad for my long-term health, and I wanted to get off it as soon as possible. So after a few weeks, with Joann's guidance, I tapered down my daily dose from 30 milligrams, to 20, to 10, but somewhere between 10 and 5 milligrams, my lung problems started up again, and the rash came back. "We've got to bump it back up," Joann said, so we increased the dose to 20 milligrams and held it there for a couple of weeks. No problems. Then we went back down to 15, then 10, and by the time we got to 5 milligrams, the reactions returned.

Throughout the fall of 2002, I went through this frustrating cycle—prednisone on, allergies off; prednisone off, allergies on. I continued to have my blood drawn every couple of weeks, and the tests showed that my white blood cell count continued to rise through November, when it peaked at about 10,000. Finally, in December, my count started dropping back down and looked like it was going to stabilize somewhere around 4,000 or 5,000. "Okay," I said to Joann, thinking back to our theory, "I think I'll be able to go completely off prednisone this time without having my horrible allergies return, because my white count is stabilizing and my nonlinear system is no longer out of whack." Terry and I were about to go to Mexico with my son Adam and his girlfriend, and Joann thought I should play it safe while there, tapering down to 10 milligrams, but not going below it. I did a very slow taper, had no troubles in Mexico, and had a wonderful trip, spending time with Adam, visiting Mayan ruins, snorkeling, and birdwatching.

As soon as I came back, I went down to 8 milligrams a day of prednisone. Still no problems. After three more days, I went down to 6 milligrams, and still no wheezing. I went to 5 milligrams. No wheezing. By the first week of January 2003, I went to zero. No allergies. I got a blood test shortly thereafter, which showed that my white count had stabilized at 5,500. "Maybe our theory wasn't so crazy after all!" I told Joann. "Yeah, it seems perfectly reasonable, but of course, one patient's experience isn't going to convince the medical world that this threshold exceedence idea will hold true for all patients. I will discuss it with my colleagues, though, and see what they think. We have all your data, and we really should write a paper on it. One of these days, I want to get around to that."

My broncospasms returned only once, for about one month after a horrible flu, but my leg allergies come and go. They're not as bad as before, but from time to time I still have to use steroid ointments to keep the rash under control. It may be an unusual side effect of the bone marrow transplant, but it's a "minor morbidity" that I gladly accept given the macabre alternative. More recently, I have been controlling the lower leg problems with compression, knee-high socks—and this home remedy that Terry pushed me to try is working! But before that, there were more problems yet to come.

CHAPTER
16 | Size Matters

AROUND THE SAME TIME my allergic dermatitis was at its worst, in November 2002, I went into the cancer center for another PCR test. The nurse took a small vial of my blood, only a few cc's, I guessed, and it was sent off to the PCR lab. After waiting anxiously for three weeks, the results came back negative, which was really great, but for some reason, my left brain was not satisfied. "What's bothering you?" Terry asked. "I've been thinking about this. Suppose only a few cancer cells survived chemo, radiation, and the bone marrow transplant, maybe in my reinjected stem cell fluid. We never PCR'ed it before the reinjection, so maybe a few malignant cells were reinjected and are hiding out in some lymph node or in a nonirradiated piece of marrow. I'm wondering how much of my blood we would have to sample to be able to detect a really low level of cancer cells." Terry told me to figure out my blood volume and divide that by the number of cancer cells I thought I might have, and see what I came up with. "How much blood do you think I have?" I asked Terry. "I don't know," Terry said, "maybe 10,000 cc's?" To keep the calculation simple, I supposed I had 10,000 cc's of blood and 1,000 cancer cells. If those 1,000 cancer cells were uniformly distributed in my blood, the probability that we'd get a positive detection of cancer doing PCR on only 1 cc of blood would be one tenth (1,000 divided by 10,000), or 10 percent, meaning the probability of a false negative (that is, finding that I was free of cancer cells when I wasn't) would be nine-tenths, or 90 percent. "I follow you so far," Terry said. I continued, "The problem is that they only PCR'ed a couple cc's of my blood, so our celebrating over my not having any cancer cells could've been premature. Maybe what we should be doing is having them take 10 cc's of blood each time, which would significantly reduce the probability of a false negative, and then see if I still have a zero cancer cell count."

I typed my latest proposal up in an e-mail and sent it to Sandra. She wrote back, telling me she wasn't sure if the sample size made any difference, but that if I really wanted 10 cc's tested, it was fine with her. So the next PCR test, which was around January 2003, was done on 10 cc's of my blood. I was scheduled to see Sandra two months later, but I knew it only took about two weeks to get the results, so after two weeks, I sent Sandra an e-mail asking her what happened with my last test. No answer. Two weeks later, I e-mailed and asked again, and she replied that she'd have to check with the lab. I was immediately suspicious. Two weeks later, Terry sent Sandra an e-mail saying, "This is driving Steve crazy. Can you please tell us what's going on?" "I need to discuss it with him personally," she wrote back, "and he's coming in next week. We'll talk about it then." My heart sank. I knew it couldn't be good news if she wouldn't tell me over e-mail.

Return of the 500-Pound Gorilla?

We waited nervously for my next appointment with Sandra, and when we saw her, the first thing she asked was, "Why were you telling me that we should take 10 cc's of blood?" I explained the whole business about having a 10 percent chance of cancer detection and a 90 percent chance of a false negative if 1 cc of blood was PCR'ed (assuming I had 1,000 cancer cells and 10,000 cc's of blood), but a much lower chance of a false negative—around 11 percent, I calculated—if 10 cc's were PCR'ed. "Well, usually, if cancer's in the blood, there's so much of it there that it doesn't matter whether you take 1 or 10 cc's, but it's true: If it were a very, very low number of cells, then you'd need a larger sample," Sandra said. I asked her what happened with my latest PCR. "The reason I did not tell you over the phone or e-mail is because I need to explain to you that we don't know what any of this means." "What any of what means?" "You had seventy-eight cancer cells per microgram of DNA—but don't forget that your cancer count was 200,000 in your bone marrow fluid and 800,000 in your lymph node when you were diagnosed. Seventy-eight is nothing. This is a very low number." Sandra's words of encouragement didn't matter; I was disconsolate. I felt like I had wrestled with a 500-pound gorilla, and it had smashed my face, broken my bones, and ripped open my skin, but I had knocked it out. Just when I thought I'd won the fight, the damn gorilla got up on the count of nine, and I didn't know how I was going to wrestle with it again.

I began arguing for maintenance therapy with Rituxan again, not wanting my cancer cells to double every month so that in another year they'd be back to 200,000. Sandra correctly pointed out that I was overreacting, as the seventy-eight figure was no indication that my cancer was growing. We'd have to track the count over time to look for any indication of multiplication. I feared that the clonal nature of cancer guaranteed that the cells would multiply, but Sandra countered that in her research, she'd found that people who had been in remission for ten or fifteen years still had positive PCRs, with low numbers like mine bouncing around, and they never got full-fledged cancer again. Apparently, their own immunities—their killer T cells—were keeping the cancer in check. I pondered this for a moment and then said, "Well, how come my cancer ever went out of control in the first place?" She explained that maybe my defenses had broken down, and I tried to visualize the process. "The cancer cells were like the members of a football team, just a bunch of clones who ran the same offensive play over and over again, scoring only when the defense was injured, asleep at the wheel, or otherwise not vigilant." Sandra laughed at my analogy but said that it was as good a theory of cancer as many.

She went on to tell me a story about a poor girl who needed a kidney, was donated one by her father, and died of melanoma six months later. Then it dawned on the family that the father had had melanoma twelve years earlier and was declared "cured," because melanoma is the kind of cancer that is typically considered gone if it doesn't come back in five years. Apparently, the father had been walking around for years with a low level of cancer cells present in his body, and while it didn't affect him—presumably because it was controlled by his own immune defenses—it did, tragically, hurt his daughter. Sandra said, "It's a horrible story, but it could be good news for you, because it shows that a person's defenses can be in control of a very low level of cancer. In fact, it is possible that everybody has a very low number of cancer cells all the time; the key is to make sure your body's natural defenses continue fighting them." "Okay," I said, "let's do another PCR test soon to see if my defenses are doing their job." Sandra recommended that I come back in three months, but I didn't want to wait that long if I had cancer cells growing exponentially inside me, so we agreed on eight weeks.

Test Result Roller Coaster

Eight weeks later, we went to Sandra's office, where the nurses took another 10 cc's of my blood, although I admit that if I really had seventy-eight cancer cells per microgram of DNA, the sample size didn't matter any more, and 1 cc would have been sufficient. After three excruciatingly long weeks, Terry and I went back to see Sandra, and she said, "Good news. It's forty-nine." She gave me an I-told-you-so look that I was thrilled to receive. "I guess going from seventy-eight to forty-nine can't be considered exponential growth," I joked. "Not at all, so let's just check it every three months from here on out and see what happens." Then I asked her the dreaded question: "Sandra, what are we going to do if it goes up?" "Well, we don't really know what a dangerous number is." I said, "Yes we do. We know that 100,000 is dangerous, and therefore, 10,000 is probably dangerous, and even 1,000 probably means that more rapid growth is occurring, so I'm going to guess that anything over 100 is bad." Sandra reminded me that we didn't have any data to back up my theories, and she was right, but I still wanted to know what we'd do if the next count was, say, 250. If the PCR showed that my cancer cell count was up to several hundred the next time and it consistently increased in subsequent tests, Sandra and I agreed that we'd treat it with Rituxan and see if we could knock it out. I suggested that if we did get as far as using Rituxan, we'd be able to track my progress by continuing to do the PCR tests on my blood, and Sandra agreed again. She mentioned that there were some emerging studies out there suggesting that maintenance therapy combined with PCR testing was effective.

If all else failed, Sandra said we could try an allo transplant or radioimmunotherapy[1] or any of a number of other new treatments that were being developed. I feebly insisted, "But wouldn't it be better just to knock it out while the count is low?" but Sandra wasn't keen on treating something that wasn't necessarily a problem. Despite that difference in opinion, we'd made enormous progress, having gotten the PCR tests and made an agreement about maintenance therapy if my counts showed a clear upward trend. I was satisfied enough by the outcome of our discussion and my latest PCR results that I agreed to wait three months for the next PCR test. (Remember, most patients in my situation would have only a CT scan as a follow-up and thus would receive treatment for recurring cancer only if large enough lumps showed up in the pictures, and thus large amounts of cancer were present.)

Three months later, I gave another 10 cc's of blood, waited the interminable three weeks, returned to Sandra's office, and was greeted by the Fellow, who matter-of-factly said, "It's fine. It's 101." I said, "It's what?!?" "101." That sounded like growth to me, so I resorted to my Rituxan argument. The Fellow promptly quashed it. "You're still in full remission, your cancer counts are nowhere near the level that they were, and you don't know that they're multiplying. A 100 count could just be noise. We warned you that we have no data on this for mantle cell; you're the experiment."

Sandra entered at that point in our discussion. We went over the PCR results again, and we agreed that if the next PCR showed that my cancer count was up substantially, we would seriously consider maintenance treatment. "I sure hope it's zero," I said. "So do I, but let's not expect *too* much."

Three months later, we repeated the routine. I had another 10 cc's of blood drawn, but had to wait only a week this time for my appointment with Sandra—or so I thought. Two days before the appointment, I got a phone call from Sandra's assistant, who informed me that Sandra had to attend a major committee meeting out of town the week of my appointment, so we'd have to reschedule. "Okay," I said, knowing I had no choice in the matter. "Could you just tell me my PCR results?" "I'm not a doctor; I can't discuss those results. Only the doctor can tell you."

Several days later, Sandra's assistant e-mailed me to say that it made no sense to have an appointment the following week. The lab that performed the PCR test was moving, and it turned out that although the technicians had run my sample, the machine was packed up before they got the quantitative results on it. It would be a few more weeks before the machine would be unpacked and I could get my results. What luck.

Hanging around waiting for the machine to be relocated and unpacked was agonizing. The longer the wait became, the more my suspicions grew, because the last time my results were delayed was when they were bad. I had these paranoid visions of my cancer count rising to 300 cells per microgram of DNA and of Sandra and her staff having a big debate about whether to treat me with Rituxan.

A week or two later, I got another e-mail from Sandra's assistant, who scheduled me to see Sandra a few days later. I wrote back and asked if Sandra would have the PCR results, and the assistant confirmed that Sandra would (but of course, I couldn't get them via e-mail). My anxiety built. Had the gorilla been knocked out, or was it slowly rebuilding its strength for the next attack? Would maintenance therapy really work if it came down to that? I wondered whether I would spend the rest of my life oscillating between remission and full-blown cancer.

By the time my appointment with Sandra rolled around, I was worried sick. I walked into her office with sweaty palms and was surprised to see there was a new Fellow. It turns out that Sandra's previous Fellow had been hired by Genentech, the manufacturer of Rituxan, as a staff scientist. I was happy for him and had no doubt that he'd do a spectacular job, as he is very knowledgeable, even if conservative in the absence of data. The new Fellow introduced himself and told me what a pleasure it was to meet me. I tried to make small talk, but I couldn't stand it any longer. I said, "Please, can you just tell me the PCR results?" "Oh, very good," he said. "Twenty." "Twenty?" I repeated, feeling as if two tons of bricks had just been lifted off my shoulders. "Twenty? Didn't Sandra say that that's the cancer count detected [via PCR] on the tonsil of someone who had a tonsillectomy but had never had cancer?" "I don't know about that," he said, "but twenty is not distinguishable from zero."

Borrowing Trouble

Terry likes to tell me when I get in my worry-wart moods that I shouldn't "borrow trouble." We knew what would have to be done if my cancer count started growing again, and there was no reason for unnecessary angst, especially since it could create stress hormones that could hurt my killer T cells, which I presumed I needed to fight my cancer. Terry was once again right. "Twenty," I said to her. "I can hardly believe it! The best I was hoping for was fifty." But in my heart of hearts, I would've loved a zero. "I wonder if I'd had a few doses of Rituxan over the past six months if I'd be at zero right now," I said. Terry smiled and said, "Yeah, me too."

When Sandra came in, she apologized for the delays and the reschedulings, but she also knew that I understood, better than almost anyone else she treated, what the life of a professor was like. "I know the pressures on you," I said, "but it doesn't stop me from nearly having an anxiety attack when I have long delays between test and results. The results were worth the wait, but I wish I'd known sooner. The last four weeks have been torture!" Sandra didn't apologize but repeated Terry's logic: "We have a plan. You don't need to be worried; things are working out really well. I hope that you'll be satisfied enough with this number that we can wait four months now until the next PCR. You're not in any danger of exponential growth or of getting your cancer back anytime soon." "I know, Sandra, I agree, but I still wish we could knock it to zero."

CHAPTER

17 | "In Cancer, Perfect

Is Important"

I AM WRITING THIS CHAPTER on an airplane in December 2003, after spending two weeks in Milan, where Terry and I attended a Conference of the Parties, a meeting of nations involved in the United Nations Framework Convention on Climate Change. There was relatively low drama at this conference compared with, say, the plenary meeting in Geneva I described earlier. By the time of the Milan meeting, there had been such violent disagreement over the Kyoto Protocol that the chances of its going into effect had been severely diminished, and people were simply getting exhausted. So the conference was a depressing event. Terry and I wandered around, picking up anti-U.S. vibes everywhere. Nobody was angry at us personally—they knew how long and hard we had been fighting with our own government to try to get a rational climate policy past the Bush administration "climate monkeys," who "see no climate, hear no climate, speak no climate." But at that point most of us agreed that no action would be taken on climate change in the United States until the administration had a dramatic change of heart or left office.

Two Kinds of Remission

Another one of the reasons we went to Milan was to visit a renowned oncologist who practices there. In her tireless search for more information, Terry had found an article in the medical journal *Blood* about a lengthy study of mantle cell lymphoma that had been done by that oncologist and about a dozen other European doctors. The doctors claimed that the protocol they used to treat patients with mantle cell lymphoma produced results that were superior to all other known protocols up to that point. Their technique seemed fairly standard: They administered chemotherapy and radiation treatment, extracted the patient's stem cells, and then eventually performed the autologous stem cell transplant, reinjecting the stem cells back into the patient's body. (This was the same type of transplant I had had.) The main difference between their protocol and others, including the one used on me, was that the European doctors went to great lengths to ensure that the patients' extracted stem cells were completely free of cancer cells before reinjecting them. After multiple chemos with a Rituxan component and radiation treatment, the doctors sampled a patient's stem cell fluid and performed a PCR test on it, to be as sure as possible that it was cancer free. If the PCR showed that cancer cells were still present, the doctors would do more chemos and then another PCR, repeating the process as many times as necessary to get the stem cell fluid clean. Then the autologous transplant would be done, and six months after the transplant, the team would extract blood from the patient and use PCR to determine whether there were still a few cancer cells floating around or whether the remission was complete. They called it "molecular remission" when the PCR test returned a zero count at that stage and "clinical remission" or "minimal residual disease" when the test reported a very low count—like my own—that basically wasn't detectable by any technique other than PCR.

I was frustrated at my inability to get a PCR test done on my stem cell fluid *before* my own autologous transplant, and to this day, I don't know whether or not residual cancer cells were present in my reinjected fluid or whether having PCR before my transplant would have improved my outcome. On the other hand, my treatment wasn't standard, either; at least I was able to get my stem cells purged with the Isolex 300i machine and to get PCR *after* my bone marrow transplant. Overall, my outcome had been very good compared with that of many others. Either way, I was interested in what these European doctors had to say and what their experiences had been with PCR-reported cancer cell counts in patients like me who were in clinical remission.

On one of our last couple days in Italy, Terry and I met with Dr. Alessandro Gianni, the lead author of the study, in his office at the Milan Cancer Center. I felt exceedingly lucky that Dr. Gianni was willing to see us while we were in town, even though we gave him short notice. Before we left the States, I had e-mailed Sandra to let her know that we were going to see Dr. Gianni, not for a second opinion, but to find out about his treatment protocol. I wanted to pick his brain about PCR results and maintenance therapy. Sandra wrote back and said, "Yes, you should see him. He's a very intriguing guy. Last week, I was at a cancer meeting in Monaco and got to meet him. I'm sure you'll be interested in what he has to say." Any cancer doc who earned Sandra's respect was definitely of interest to me.

Dr. Gianni began our meeting by explaining his work and giving a simple summary of the findings presented in his paper in *Blood*. He and his team had compared the remission rates achieved with his protocol with those obtained with different protocols that they had tracked since the mid-1980s. The difference in results was dramatic. After five years, about 80 percent of Dr. Gianni's patients were still in their original remissions, and those who were not had had PCR results showing cancer cells in their reinjected stem cell fluid. The remission rates for his control group (patients who underwent more conventional treatments, such as CHOP, without

PCR testing) were much lower; after five years, more than 50 percent of them had lost remission. That made us very uneasy. However, after reading Dr. Gianni's paper carefully on the flight to Milan, I realized that his control group, patients who did not have PCR done on their stem cell fluid prior to reinjection, had not had *my* treatment either; that is, they had not had CHOP *plus* Rituxan, let alone the use of the Isolex 300i stem-cell-cleansing machine. Therefore, it occurred to me that I couldn't be compared with either his test group or his control group. (I also realized that until more frequency data on patients like myself and those in Dr. Gianni's test group were available, it would be nearly impossible to determine what elements of treatment were most essential to the positive results. Was it the PCR? The Isolex? The Rituxan? Or was it all these things in combination?)

We brought this up after explaining my treatment. "You're absolutely right that you had a much better treatment than the people in our control group, but perhaps not as good as the ones who were in our test group," he said. "It will be very difficult to compare you with our test group anyway, as there were only twenty-seven patients in our study, and they were spread across multiple European centers. There's still not a lot of data . . ." I interrupted to say that Sandra didn't have many more patients in her own studies, and he said, "Exactly. That's why most of what we'll do is intuitive and involves subjectivity, not just the perusal of clinical trials databases." I knew right away why Sandra said I was going to like this doctor.

A True Zero

Dr. Gianni then asked to see my PCR results. We showed him the 800,000 per microgram of DNA from the PCR on the cancerous lymph node; the 200,000 from the 40 percent cancer-infected bone marrow fluid (both before my treatments); the zero count from the bone marrow biopsy done three or four months after the transplant; the zero for the first two PCRs, done on only a couple of cc's of blood; then the 78, the 49, and the 101; and finally, the good news, the recent 20. "What do you think the last few PCR values mean?" he asked us. "I don't know. We have been told that they're not statistically different from zero, but they're still not zero." He fully agreed, repeating Sandra's line that we still didn't know enough about PCR in this context to have a definitive answer as to what concentration of cancer cells separated a dangerous level from background-level noise. However, Dr. Gianni thought that noise was probably around 20 or 30, since PCRs done on the tissue of healthy people who had never had cancer resulted in values in that range. But did that mean my PCR result of 101 was evidence of residual cancer?

Now my PCR results were back down to twenty cancer cells per microgram of DNA, and at that level I could very well live the rest of my life in remission, with my immunities keeping the background cancer in check. But what if those twenty cells per microgram *were* active and the cancer made a comeback? Was it prudent to ignore the low counts, doing nothing while the cancer cells could be multiplying and attempting to give me a full-fledged disease again? Dr. Gianni didn't think so. Hearing him say this was music to my ears, although it was stressful to think that I'd have to whip out my old maintenance therapy argument when I returned home and saw Sandra.

To reinforce his point and give me some ammunition to use when back at Stanford, Dr. Gianni said, "Let's do a cost-benefit analysis without worrying about the financial costs of the treatment [about $15,000 per bottle of Rituxan]. Let's talk about the health trade-offs only. What are the benefits of maintenance therapy using Rituxan? Let's say you need six treatments or so over the next eight months." "I don't know," I said. "Perhaps we'd eliminate all my remaining cancer cells while there are so few of them.

Maintenance therapy might drive it down to a true zero." "Yes, it might do that—or it might not. We are still unsure of how and whether Rituxan works for maintenance therapy. What are the costs?" I said, "Well, Sandra was worried that if I had any aberrant B cells that didn't have CD-20 receptors, we might induce them to become much more aggressive than they would be otherwise, and then they would not be treatable with Rituxan, but she didn't think there was a high probability of that, nor did Ron Levy." "Nor do I," he said. "I can't absolutely rule that out as a risk, but is living with a number of cancer cells, although exceedingly low and indistinguishable from zero, and knowing that they might turn into statistically significant numbers in the future, worth the risk? What is the real cost of trying to get rid of them?" "We've been arguing that way for the last two years!" Terry exclaimed. "We finally reached an agreement with Sandra that if the numbers start to climb, we'll treat the cancer with Rituxan." "Why wait? Why not just knock it out if you can now? That's what I'd do with a patient with your numbers—and it's what I'd do for myself if I was in your situation. Your result, while excellent, is not perfect, and in cancer, perfect is important."

Dr. Gianni then launched into a discussion of type I versus type II errors, another topic familiar from the climate change debate. Again, a type I error involves accepting and acting on a forecast that turns out to be false, and a type II error involves rejecting or ignoring a forecast that proves to be true. With my cancer, the type I error would be to do maintenance therapy right away and later find out (though I'm not sure how) that since my cancer cell counts were not statistically different from zero, the cancer never would have come back, and there had been no need to attack the low level of cancer cells with Rituxan again. Then only the financial costs of the treatment and any small chance of negative physical side effects would be the cost of this error. The type II error, on the other hand, could be deadly. We would be committing a type II error if, because of uncertainties and lack of clinical trials data, we decided against the Rituxan maintenance therapy, and my low numbers of cancer cells multiplied exponentially until I had full-fledged cancer again. And this was assuming that the Rituxan would work, which was in itself not a certainty but a plausible inference based on process knowledge.

I asked Dr. Gianni why it was so much easier for patients in Europe to get PCR, even before their stem cell fluid had been reinjected in the transplant. I had recently spoken with a friend in France who was also battling cancer, and he mentioned that the first time he asked for PCR, his doctor agreed to have it done. Dr. Gianni thought that the French doctor's willingness to have PCR done on his patient was not simply because European doctors are more open to trying new techniques for which little data is available, but because the health care system is structured differently in many European nations than it is in the United States. Because medical care in France and other European countries is paid for by the state rather than by private insurance companies, there is less hesitation to perform expensive tests and procedures, especially in cancer treatment. *That's great*, I thought, *but how is it going to help me?*

After about an hour, our cancer conversation was over, and Dr. Gianni switched gears, asking why we were in Milan. We told him about the conference, and it turned out that he had a very deep and abiding interest in climate change, so we spent another twenty minutes chatting about that. I told him I thought the type I versus type II error problem was the same with climate change. If governments resorted to the precautionary principle in dealing with climate change and acted immediately to curb it, they'd commit a type I error if their worries about climate change proved to be unfounded and our emissions didn't greatly modify the climate. The time, money, and other resources spent to adapt to or prevent climate change would have been wasted, or at least could have been put to better use tackling other environmental or social problems. The type II error would occur if drastic climate change did happen and proved to be destructive, yet no hedging actions had been taken because uncertainty was used as an excuse to delay policy. In both cancer and climate, I preferred not to risk the type II error, and Dr. Gianni wholeheartedly agreed.

We left, thanking Dr. Gianni warmly for giving us an hour and a half of his time and telling him how much we appreciated his philosophy. I tried to calm my own fears, which had been reignited by our discussion, by saying: "I don't have to panic about this, given that my numbers are so low. We could take some time to work out what to do." "Absolutely right," he said. "This is not an issue of deep urgency because you are likely to remain in this kind of remission for the foreseeable future, but if there's very little health cost, why not try to get rid of every last vestige you may have of this very nasty disease?" I agreed, realizing that if Dr. Gianni were a climatologist, our views on policy actions would probably be identical.

Same Argument, Different Day

In January 2004, Terry and I had an appointment with Sandra to discuss our meeting with Dr. Gianni and to get the numbers from my latest PCR test. "So what did Alessandro say?" Sandra asked, about thirty seconds after telling us my latest PCR was a disturbing (to me) 122. "He said that were it he with my PCR results, he wouldn't wait for 'definitive proof' of residual cancer via escalating PCR counts but would treat it right away with maintenance therapy using Rituxan." "Well, were it I with your cancer, I'd wait to be sure I needed the treatments," Sandra said, and I feared we were launching into another stalemate. "But I fully agree that we should do maintenance therapy if it ever seems like the cancer is returning." "But why take the risk and wait? The cost of a type II error is too high to ignore." "Because I don't fully agree that Rituxan carries no health risks," she replied. "Rituxan is not nearly as threatening as the CHOP chemicals, but it does force your body to kill off your B cells, and you need them for infection fighting. Immunodepression is definitely a cost we have to consider." So in this case, there *was* a health cost—or at least a reasonable chance of a health cost—if a type I error was committed.

I mentioned a remark Ron Levy had made in a video available on his Web site about the need for maintenance therapy. "Why not ask him?" Sandra said. She stepped out for about ten minutes, and, to our delight, returned with Ron Levy in tow. So, we asked him, "Aren't you in favor of maintenance therapy?" "Yes, but . . . " "But what?" "I don't think your PCR tests reveal anything other than that you are dramatically better than you were. We simply can't distinguish 20 from 80 from 122 from zero [he had obviously seen the new numbers]. I agree with Sandra that the Rituxan could possibly have negative side effects, and we don't want to use it if it's not necessary. If we stay vigilant with the PCRs and we see a significant and systematic increase over the next few tests, *then* you should go ahead with the Rituxan therapy. That will still be well before your cancer could ever be detected in a CT scan." "Can I get this next PCR test in two months instead of four?" "Fair enough," Sandra said. Terry and I looked at each other and accepted that compromise—we now realized that there was some risk to Rituxan maintenance therapy that we hadn't fully appreciated.

I was pleased by the new compromise we struck with Sandra, but not entirely satisfied. Lodged in a deep, dark corner of my mind was the question of why my PCR results had been zero for the nine months after my bone marrow transplant and had not been zero since. Was it really due to a larger sample size (going from testing a few cc's to 10 cc's of blood), or were my cancer cells actually multiplying? Or was there a third explanation we hadn't even imagined? Our agreed-on plan simply to monitor my cancer cell trends seemed the best strategy at that moment. But for how long?

I couldn't help but think that if Terry and I hadn't taken the initiative and pushed the system, asking others to consider our logic, this discussion may not have happened, given the megabusy lives of cancer pioneers like Sandra Horning and Ron Levy. It is yet another example of why patients from hell—or even less aggressive patients and their advocates—can help improve their treatments and convince doctors to focus on the best strategies for each individual, which could spill over and benefit many other patients as well.

CHAPTER

18 | "I Think Your Kidneys
Did You a Favor"

The Next Three Years

Earlier on, a few days of my life took up a chapter, but now, I'll squeeze three years into a single one.

As Karl Blume predicted, my system was out of balance for at least a year after my bone marrow transplant, and the side effects, while not fatal, were certainly highly annoying. Fortunately, I saw the last of my allergic reactions in January 2003, and by that time the edema had also calmed down, for a while at least. My primary worries then shifted to getting my full energy back and getting the neuropathy in my feet under control so that I could do outdoor activities without the risk of injuring myself as a result of my lack of dexterity. I checked in with Sandra every three months to get a PCR test and doggedly pestered her about getting Rituxan as a preventive maintenance therapy, particularly since in our Web research we'd seen reports that preliminary studies performed in a few far-flung places were finally showing that the strategy was proving to be effective in patients.

A massively heavy travel schedule for work, along with holidays in Australia, Papua New Guinea, New Caledonia, and other places, made 2003 a fabulous year. I found that I could still hike, one of my favorite vacation pastimes, if I used a walking stick, which at least partially compensated for the pain and clumsiness caused by the peripheral neuropathy in my feet. I got winded very easily when climbing up even small hills, a frustration I still have to this day, though it has improved substantially since I got an athletic trainer and have been working out.

Just a Flu Bug?

In November 2003, more and new trouble started. I went to Boston to meet with my colleagues from the Ecological Society of America and the Boston Aquarium to select twenty scientists for the highly esteemed Aldo Leopold Leadership program. This program takes ecologists and a few other scientists, typically in mid-career, and trains them in leadership and effectiveness. They learn how to communicate with the media, how to talk to members of Congress, how to interact with representatives of the business community and address their concerns, and other methods of making science accessible to the public, skills about which most scientists are abysmally ignorant.

I boarded the plane to Boston with a slight sore throat and a mild cold, one of the few I had had despite still being slightly immunocompromised. By the time I got to my hotel, my slight cold had morphed into a raging flu. My temperature went up over 102, which prompted me to call Mike Jacobs, my internist. "It sounds like the flu," he said. "But I got a flu shot." "The flu shot missed some really significant strains this year, so you probably got a variety not covered by it," Mike said. "Do you have an antibiotic with you?" "Yes, I always travel with Zithromax." "Take it," he said. "I don't think you have a bacterial infection, but given your situation, and that you're on the road, you don't want to risk developing one, particularly in your lungs, so just take it prophylactically. Come home as soon as you're able."

I felt very guilty and depressed about not being able to attend the Leopold Fellowship meeting, especially since I had spent so much time reading up on each of the candidates. But a fever was a fever, and coming to the meeting sick wouldn't have been fair or polite to others, something I had learned after being immunocompromised for so long myself. So I called Jane Lubchenco, the chair of the program, and explained my situation. Jane still wanted me to participate, so she arranged to have a speakerphone at the meeting. The next day, I called in to the meeting from my hotel room, and for eight hours that day, I lay in bed, not feeling too great, taking Tylenol to keep my fever down, drinking tea, and working with the committee over the phone. We made good progress, and at the end of the day, my colleagues announced that they were rewarding themselves with a trip to a wonderful seafood restaurant while I stayed in bed miserable. I was disappointed that I couldn't attend the social outing but was glad that I was still able to make a contribution to the candidate selection process. At least I didn't do all that reading for nothing, nor did I disappoint my colleagues by not participating.

On the second day of the meeting, I felt better, though still pretty sick, so I popped a few more Tylenol, got my fever under 100, hurried to the airport, and flew home while flying was still possible. I regretted missing the second and final day of the meeting, but if you've ever been sick and stranded far from home, I'm sure you can appreciate the urgency I felt.

It wasn't a fun trip. I was very careful to wear my mask throughout the flight because I didn't want to infect anybody else, and I cleaned my hands frequently with alcohol lotion so as not to spread germs that way. In addition to the misery caused by the flu bug, I noticed yet another annoying malady: My legs were unusually swollen, and I had to get up regularly and walk around the plane to prevent further swelling. When I lifted my legs with each step or even just jiggled them while sitting, I could actually feel fluid sloshing from my calves to my hamstrings. I chalked that up to being tired and sick and drinking too much tea, and I tried to ignore it.

About a week later, the flu ended, but the edema did not. I let Sandra and her team know about it, but they didn't seem particularly interested, since the edema was annoying, not life threatening, and was probably just a recurring side effect of my treatment. In any case, my latest PCR was a nice low number—around thirty—and they thought I was doing just great.

"What Are You Looking For?"

Mike Jacobs was more concerned. "I don't like it," he responded when I called him about the edema. "Come in for some tests." He ordered a urine test, which, to my recollection, I had never had in all the time I spent in the hospital and doctors' offices in the previous few years. He also ordered some blood protein tests, which I had had before. They had come back normal the first time around, so I wondered what could have changed over a relatively short period of time. "What are you looking for, Michael?" I asked. "I want to see how your kidneys are doing," he said, "because this sounds a little bit like nephrotic syndrome. The blood and urine tests will let us know." "Is that bad?" I asked. "Not necessarily. It depends on how severe it is and what caused it, though it's difficult to figure out causation in many cases."

A day after my tests, Mike called to tell me that my protein numbers weren't too good but weren't in any way life threatening. He wanted me to see a colleague of his in the nephrology department at Stanford. The nephrology unit is home to the doctors who deal with dialysis, transplants, and other kidney-related procedures. I made an appointment with Dr. Jeff Petersen, who is Professor of Medicine (nephrology), and went in to see him.

On arriving at the nephrology unit for my appointment, Terry and I were met by Dr. Petersen's very impressive young Fellow, Luis Alvarez, and we spent quite a bit of time discussing nephrotic

syndrome with him. Unlike the young oncologists, who'd been relatively unconcerned about my edema, Luis listened to my story
and looked at my recent blood and urine tests with a furrowed
brow. He was sure that the tremendous excess of protein in my
urine and the substantial deficit in my blood were causing the
edema. The low protein level in my blood was allowing fluids to
leak from my blood vessels and into the tissue in my legs and arms,
making them swell. Luis was worried not just because my protein
levels were completely imbalanced but because the blood and
urine tests performed the day I visited nephrology showed a
degradation in my condition by about a factor of two compared
with the tests Mike Jacobs had ordered a week or so earlier. "I
think we need to take this quite seriously and pursue rigorous
treatment immediately," Luis said, and when his mentor arrived
fifteen minutes later, a slightly different version of the same message came through.

Luis, a very nice young man, was nonetheless honest and direct,
a characteristic I would expect in any good scientist. "Nobody
knows for certain what causes nephrotic syndrome, but we do
know that the numbers you have now, if left unchecked, could,
over the course of a year or two, deteriorate significantly and lead
to kidney failure, something I'm certain you do not want." That
was quite a shock, and it obviously got my attention. I told Jeff and
Luis to order whatever tests they thought necessary and was much
more willing to undergo more poking and prodding than I might
have been otherwise.

Jeff and Luis ordered two tests: a kidney biopsy and a
colonoscopy. I could understand the kidney biopsy (though I must
admit, the last thing I really wanted was a pin stuck in my kidneys), because my kidneys were the problem, but why the
colonoscopy? I asked Jeff about it, and he said, "Well, sometimes
cancers create proteins that coat the kidney and are released into
the colon, where they can create the symptoms you're having.
Doing a colonoscopy will allow us to look for these proteins and

any other abnormal conditions." "But I had a CT scan less than a year ago; wouldn't that have shown cancer of the magnitude you're describing?" "It may have grown back since the CT scan." "But I *know* my cancer count is astronomically low because I had a PCR test just a few weeks ago, and the numbers were 10,000 times smaller than when I was acutely sick." "It may not take that much cancer to generate some of these proteins that can cause trouble, so let's do the colonoscopy to rule it out."

Mike Jacobs recommended an endoscopist for the colonoscopy, and I went and had the test. "Are you using Versed?" I asked. "Yessir," was the answer. "Do you need me to move around or do anything?" "Nope." "Then give me all you can give," I joked back, and they did, for the next thing I remembered was waking up saying, "When are you going to do it?" They let me know the procedure was over and everything went fine. They also mentioned that they decided to take some biopsy specimens of my colon just to see if there was any cancer hiding there. "There won't be," I said adamantly, "because I just had a PCR and I know my cancer cell counts are low." "Well, just in case. It isn't the only cancer that's possible, you know," the endoscopist replied.

Needless to say, I was very uneasy in the week before I got the biopsy results. Finally, they came back and were—wouldn't you know it—inconclusive. "There were too many B cells in your ileum," the report said, "but microscopic examination revealed no obvious cancer cells." So the ileum cells were sent to another lab for other tests, and after two distressing weeks of waiting, it turned out that the lab was unable to perform the tests because the cells in the sample had already aged too much.

Sandra Horning, on hearing about the visit to the nephrologists, the colonoscopy, and the ileum biopsy, said, "I wish they wouldn't do these kinds of tests, because even if they found some small number of cancer cells in your ileum tissue, we wouldn't know what to do about it." "Maintenance therapy," I answered automatically. "But you'd have to know it was a B cell cancer for the maintenance therapy we've been discussing to be effective," she re-torted. "If the numbers end up being as low as your PCR numbers, there's nothing we'd want to do immediately anyway; we'd just have to monitor it."

An Unrelated Disease?

A few days after the colonoscopy, I went back in to the nephrology department to see Jeff and Luis for my kidney biopsy. "How much Versed are you going to give me, Luis?" I asked. "None," he said. "I'll need you to breathe when I say 'breathe' and turn when I say 'turn,' but I promise you it won't hurt very much. I'll give you Novocain." I said, "The bone marrow biopsy guys said it wouldn't hurt much, too, and everything was fine until the needle hit the bone." "This won't be that bad. You'll just feel some pressure and maybe a little ache; it'll be nothing like a bone marrow biopsy." I told Luis I'd try to stay calm, but I became doubly nervous when Terry wasn't allowed in the room, because that meant I wouldn't have the hand to hold that helped me get through those other horrible procedures. But I was told that there wasn't enough room for Terry, it was not the kind of thing you wanted a spouse to watch, and it wasn't that painful anyway, so I went along with it—not that there was anything I could have done about it.

Indeed, Luis was right. The kidney biopsy was not very painful. It wasn't a walk in the park, but it wasn't a fall off a cliff. Jeff and Luis took three samples, and then I had to hang around the hospital for eight hours afterward, to make certain there was no internal bleeding. I was able to go home early the next morning. Sitting in the hospital overnight brought back memories that I had blocked out of my mind until then, and they conjured up very mixed feelings—elation that two years after my clean-room experience I was still alive and had a very low cancer cell count, and fear that I still hadn't won the battle and that I had some other problem cropping up that could be really serious.

A week later, I went back to see the nephrologists. Luis confirmed that they had not found any cancer in my kidneys and that I didn't even have much scarring in my kidneys, which was surprising, given the beating they took from the chemo and the bone marrow transplant. I was relieved but knew the problem was still something serious. I waited for Luis's diagnosis. "You have membranous glomerulonephritis—MG for short." "What's that?" I asked, stumbling over the words. "Well, it's a type of nephrotic syndrome that occurs when proteins form a membrane in the glomeruli, which are some 30 million tubes in your kidneys that filter your blood and separate protein between blood and urine. The membrane in your kidneys is allowing too much protein to seep out of your blood and into your urine. Your capillary walls are leakier as a result of this lack of protein in your blood."

It sounded pretty serious, and as much as I wanted to hide from the latest diagnosis, I asked what was next. "Well, we'd like to figure out what caused the MG, but it's a very difficult disease to pin down. You had a rare lymphoma, and now you have a rare kidney syndrome, and I'm not sure they're unrelated," Luis surmised. I mentioned that I didn't think my very low number of remaining lymphoma cells could possibly be the culprit. Jeff thought they could be producing proteins that were causing trouble, or that I had graft-versus-host disease. Terry jumped in: "No, it can't be graft-versus-host disease. He had an auto transplant, not an allo." "Well, I'm glad we can scratch that one," said Jeff.

The room was silent for a moment as we all tried to think of a logical explanation for my MG. Luis broke the silence, saying, "Well, here's what we know in general about MG: About one-third of these cases just appear spontaneously and disappear spontaneously many months or years later. Another third of the cases remain at a steady state, and the last third become really bad." "Really bad?" I asked. Luis again mentioned the possibility of kidney failure, and I made it clear that I wanted to treat the MG immediately. "Well, unfortunately," said Jeff, "treatment 'by the book' means giving you cyclosporine." "Cyclosporine?" Terry and I both exclaimed simultaneously. We had learned about cyclosporine earlier in my treatment process. It was an antirejection drug that ameliorated rejection reactions by suppressing a patient's T cells. I reminded Jeff and Luis that I might have minimal residual disease and that I was still slightly immunocompromised. I needed every T cell I had to fight viruses, fend off other diseases, and keep my cancer numbers in check. Luis and Jeff fully agreed that cyclosporine was not worth the risk, so we went through the other treatment options. Prednisone sometimes worked, and Jeff thought it might be worth a shot, but he told us not to expect much.

Rituxan Again

Jeff, clearly going out on a limb, said, "Well, there's a new paper suggesting that Rituxan—you know, the monoclonal antibody you were given for your cancer—also helps people with MG." My eyes lit up. Now *that* was the best idea I'd heard yet. Jeff explained that the study reported in the paper showed that out of eight patients with MG, all of whom were given four Rituxan treatments over the course of a month, seven showed substantial improvement after a year.

"We've been trying to convince the oncologists to give Steve Rituxan as maintenance therapy for the last two years, and they keep insisting that he doesn't need it because his cancer cell numbers aren't jumping off the charts," Terry said. "Well," Jeff said, "if the prednisone doesn't work, I think you're going to get your Rituxan after all." I couldn't help but laugh: I would actually be *grateful* for the kidney problems if they led to cancer maintenance therapy with Rituxan.

I took prednisone for the next month, and the few rashes I had disappeared completely, but my edema got worse, not better. I had ten or fifteen pounds of extra fluid in my legs, which made walking and climbing stairs a chore. Every time I pressed my fingers into my leg, they left a half-inch depression that made me look like the Pillsbury Doughboy until my leg slowly reassumed its normal—if puffy—shape. My left hand was also puffy.

It was clear from the symptoms and from more blood and urine tests—good old Bayesian updating again—that the prednisone was not working, so after four weeks Jeff advised me to stop taking it. I needed another month to taper down from the 60 milligrams I had been taking, during which time Terry and I searched the Web for information on MG treatments using Rituxan. We found out that not only was Rituxan effective in abating MG in the seven of eight patients it was given to, as Jeff had mentioned, but it was also reported to have worked very well in another study of MG done in Japan.

When we went to see Sandra for our routinely scheduled appointment in oncology, she was already aware of Jeff Petersen's proposal about using Rituxan to treat my MG. She was somewhat skeptical but said she had heard it was effective for MG, though she had no idea why. I told her I thought it was the most attractive option we had left for treating the MG, and the only one that had the potential to kill two birds with one stone. However, I was a little nervous, because the nephrology department had never used Rituxan for treating MG before, and Jeff and Luis had no experience administering the drug. I asked Sandra if the oncology department would be willing to do the deed and proposed that we pick a dosage and a schedule that would serve two purposes simultaneously: helping to reduce the MG and providing maintenance therapy.

Terry gave Sandra several articles she had downloaded from the Web showing that maintenance therapy with Rituxan had been used more frequently over the past two years, and the doctors administering it were reporting that it had helped significantly in eliminating minimal residual disease in patients with B-cell lymphoma. Sandra was well aware of these new studies and even conceded that our discussions from two or three years ago, when I was told that there were no data on maintenance therapy with Rituxan, could now be replaced with a discussion about there being some data, although they were limited. Given the new data, Sandra agreed that although my cancer count was not climbing, maintenance therapy wasn't such a bad idea, especially since the nephrologists thought it would be helpful as well. I nearly shouted with joy.

So we had a deal, although Sandra cautioned me that none of the other patients she had treated before had developed MG, and she had little experience with it in that context, so we were going to be flying blind as to any clear understanding (process knowledge) of what happened after maintenance therapy. But still, I couldn't help but feel pleased. Thanks to my kidneys' glitch, Sandra and the oncologists were now willing to administer four doses of Rituxan over the course of a month—which was both the regimen used a few times for maintenance therapy and the protocol carried out in Europe on the seven patients whose Rituxan treatments for MG were successful.

A Willing Guinea Pig

When Terry and I went back to see the nephrologists, I mentioned Sandra's comment about lacking process knowledge about the effects that using Rituxan as maintenance therapy and to combat MG would have on a patient like me who had had full-blown mantle cell lymphoma. To begin gathering these data, I suggested that once the Rituxan treatments had started, we should perform tests on me every two weeks to monitor the protein in my urine and blood, and anything else Jeff and Luis thought relevant. (Sandra later added to that a test to count my CD-20 B cells—the ones that Rituxan knocks out.) Then, instead of only having endpoint data, as most clinical trials do, we'd actually know what was going on throughout the process. "You'll be the first patient ever reported this way for Rituxan and MG," Luis said, "because in the study of the eight patients, their progress was only reported at the end, after about a year." "Well, why don't you write a paper on this? You can use me for getting the information." "Okay," Luis said. "Here's a standing order for you to get blood and urine tests every two weeks. We're happy to have a willing guinea pig."

—| |—

It was with some trepidation that I went to the infusion room, now very different from the one where my chemo had been done because the cancer ward had moved to a new wing of Stanford Hospital. The new infusion room was much more pleasant, so the memories that going in for the latest round of Rituxan brought back weren't as strong as anticipated.

I remembered to tell the nurses about the horrible bout I had with Rituxan the first time I had it infused, fearing that a repeat reaction was in the cards. "We'll go very slowly," one nurse promised. "Just let us know if anything unpleasant happens." Just like the first time, three years earlier, I crept my way from 50 milligrams of Rituxan per hour to 100 milligrams per hour. After two hours, when about two-thirds of the bottle remained, I still didn't have any horrible symptoms. "Are you sure you feel completely normal?" The nurse asked. "Well, I have a bit of a scratchy throat, and my inner ear itches. It feels like the same reaction I have when I eat ripe cantaloupe." At my mention of this, the nurse immediately shut off the Rituxan drip and said she'd be back in five minutes. She came back with a supersized drip bag of Benadryl. "But you already gave me Benadryl," I protested, "and I'm so sleepy from it that I can barely keep my eyes open." "Well, we're going to make you much sleepier," she said unapologetically. "I'm going to double your dose, since I think your symptoms are the beginning of a reaction to Rituxan, and we do *not* want it to get any worse." So I got the extra double dose of Benadryl, and a double chain mail suit descended upon me. The next thing I remember was waking up feeling fine, realizing that three or four hours had passed and there was almost nothing left in the Rituxan bottle, and seeing Terry looking rather pleased with herself because she had finished a good fraction of the sweater she was knitting for a friend's child.

The first Rituxan treatment was successful, at least in terms of my not having any reactions or symptoms. As for its effects on my edema and cancer cell count, we'd just have to wait and see. About three days after the Rituxan infusion, I pressed my finger into my leg, and I thought that maybe, just maybe, the impression it made was less deep. Over the next two days, I saw further improvements. "According to my 'edema meter,' my legs are getting better," I said cheerfully to Terry. "I really think this is working."

The following week, I went in to the oncology department for Rituxan treatment number two. This time, I got a double dose of Benadryl at the outset, since the nurses remembered the slight reaction I had the previous time and didn't want to take any chances. As it turned out, I had no trouble of any kind and was finished with the infusion in less than four hours. I was tolerating the Rituxan well, although I was a little disappointed because by the time I went in for that second Rituxan infusion, the edema had pretty much gone back to where it was before we started the treatments. My protein numbers were only slightly better, but not enough to get excited about.

The nephrologists were worried that my MG was still very serious and that I should be excreting more fluid to combat it. To accomplish this, they prescribed Lasix, a diuretic often used by people with heart failure. The problem with taking diuretics isn't just that it forces you to run to the bathroom every half hour (and thus is not ideal for people who take long airplane trips or teach two-hour classes, both of which were common experiences for me), but also that they deprive your body of the electrolytes it needs to maintain normal heart rhythms, muscle control, and other bodily functions. The electrolytes are leached from the body through the frequent urination diuretics induce. I told the nephrologists that I was taking vitamin pills, which might prevent me from having problems with the diuretic. They thought the vitamins might help but warned me that I might still have trouble. However, they offered no further instructions at that time on what to do to prevent or deal with problems.

A Freeway Remedy

Three days after I started taking the diuretic, I had a lecture to give up at the California State University at Chico. Terry and I drove up to Chico the day of the lecture, and on the way there, my hands began to cramp. Near the end of the trip, the cramps were so painful that my fingers were twisted to the point that I had to pull them apart with my other fingers. The cramps moved up my hands, and soon I had pain in my wrists. I called Mike Jacobs's office from the car. He was away, but his young assistant was there, and she said, "This sounds very serious. It sounds like you have an electrolyte deficiency from the Lasix." She told me to stop at the emergency room in Chico and have them run some tests to check my electrolytes. "I have a lecture to give at 7:00 tonight and a dean to meet at 5:00. I've had these cramps on and off for the last week, though I admit they're worse today than they've been, but I'm not sure I have time for the test. Can I put it off until tomorrow?" She didn't like that answer but told me she'd check with the nephrologists and get back to me. About half an hour later, Mike's junior doc called back on my cell phone and said, "I just spoke to Luis Alvarez. He told me to tell you he *insists* that you go get an electrolyte panel done at the hospital. The docs there will know what to do to treat you. You should really try to get into the ER for treatment and then come home first thing tomorrow." I said, "Well, what are you worried about?" "Calcium and potassium deficiency. If the deficiency is sufficient, it could alter your heart rhythms, which already aren't great."

We were almost in Chico, so there was no sense in turning around and heading back home at that point. There was a hospital in Chico with an emergency room, but I didn't want to go there. I didn't want to set foot in an emergency room unless I was literally on death's doorstep. "Would you stop at the next gas station?" I asked Terry. Five minutes later, she pulled off the highway and rolled up to a gas station. I marched in, bought two chocolate milks and two bananas, walked out and said, "I'm going to take my potassium and calcium pills now." Terry smiled approvingly. I wolfed down the bananas and the chocolate milks, and Terry pulled back onto the road for the last hour of the trip to Chico.

When we arrived, my hands were still locked in painful knots. We parked on the Chico State campus, met our host, Jim Pushnik, and told him of the problem, and he took us to the emergency room at the Chico Hospital. This was the time scheduled to meet with the dean, and I felt bad that I wasn't able to do it. "Your health is more important than any dean," said Jim, "so let's get you in there."

It wasn't as easy as it sounded. When we arrived at the ER, it was immediately clear that there was no way that I was going to get out of there in less than four hours. In order to get treated, I would have had to miss my talk, which had been widely advertised and already had hundreds of people signed up to attend. "I only need a blood test," I protested to the triage nurse. "Can't I just get that and go?" "No, our rules say that you have to see a doctor first, and he has to decide on the tests you need."

I contemplated what I should do, but my hands decided for me. After about two hours in the ER, it appeared that my freeway remedy of chocolate milk and bananas was beginning to work. Slowly but surely, the cramps diminished, and eventually I felt absolutely normal. I told Terry I thought I should go ahead with the lecture. She looked at the clock nervously, noting that we only had twenty-five minutes until the lecture was supposed to begin. I walked up to the triage nurse and said, "I need this test today, but you have too many people in front of me right now. I have no symptoms any more, so I'm going to leave, give my lecture, have dinner, and come back to the ER at 10:00 p.m., when it's quieter." She said, "It's your choice, sir, but as long as you have no symptoms, I won't object." Terry, Jim, and I hustled out of the ER and made it to the lecture hall just in time. I gave my talk in a packed auditorium, had dinner and a very pleasant evening with Terry and some Chico State faculty, and by the end of the evening, the cramps were nothing but a memory. I felt it was ridiculous to go back to the ER for the calcium and potassium tests, but I'd promised Mike Jacobs's assistant I would do it, so at 10:00 p.m., we dutifully went back to the ER, and by 11:00 p.m., we were finished. Both of the tests were normal. I have been on "banana pills" ever since. No cramps, either.

The Meaning of Zero

Terry and I took a two-week trip to Argentina and Iguazu Falls in between my Rituxan treatments. Although I was supposed to get Rituxan every week for a month, I didn't see any reason to cancel the trip, because I knew full well that we were winging it with the dosage, and the docs really had no idea whether having one, two, or three weeks between rounds of Rituxan made any difference. I checked with Sandra, Jeff, and Luis, and they gave me the go-ahead. Having the treatments spread out over six weeks rather than four was irrelevant, as far as they knew.

When we returned from our trip, I went in to the oncology department for my next appointment. They had run a blood panel after the ghouling I had had during the previous appointment, and they found that my B cells with CD-20 receptors (the ones that had carried the cancer) had been wiped out by the Rituxan, but the non-CD-20 cells remained, which meant the Rituxan was working. I supposed I should have been happy that the Rituxan might be killing cancer cells and putting an end to my minimal residual disease, but in reality, I was concerned. By the time we returned from Argentina, my edema had gotten worse again, and I was back to being the Pillsbury Doughboy. *Does this mean the Rituxan isn't going to do anything for my MG?* I wondered. I asked Luis about it, and he said, "Not so fast. It takes a long time for the membranous kidney coatings characteristic of MG to disappear, so let's give this a little while." So I played out the series and went ahead with the third and fourth Rituxan treatments.

Shortly after my fourth and final Rituxan infusion, I went in to oncology for my quarterly PCR test. A week later, I went back for the results, and lo and behold, who should be there but Sean Bohen, one of Sandra's Fellows with whom we'd debated about maintenance therapy three years earlier. Sean was still employed as a researcher at Genentech, but he found that he missed practicing medicine, so he had decided to come back to Stanford Hospital part time and work a few mornings a week so that he had the opportunity to interact with real patients. It was fun to see him again, and he gave us a warm greeting.

Ironically, it was Sean—the same Sean who a few years earlier had been very skeptical of maintenance therapy—who gave us the results of my post–maintenance-therapy PCR. "Amazing!" He said. "As much as I hate to admit it, you guys were right about using Rituxan for maintenance therapy. Your PCR cancer count is now zero. I think your kidneys did you a favor." I was really impressed by Sean's frank admission. He said he'd learned a lot from my case and that everybody in the oncology department was thinking and talking about it. Terry and I were thrilled, not just because of Sean's words, but also because my cancer count was zero, and now, a month after the last Rituxan treatment, my "edema meter" had gone from high to medium. My legs were still puffy, but nothing like before.

The nephrologists weren't so sure. "Well, we'll have to see what the urine tests say," Luis said. The following week, I went in for my appointment in nephrology, and Luis confirmed that the Rituxan therapy had significantly improved my MG; I had half as much protein in my urine and twice as much in my blood as I did before the Rituxan. "You're not there yet, and in fact your numbers are still borderline for doing damage to your kidneys," Luis said, "but they're getting better. We're going to put you on a low-protein diet and see what happens."

I went on the low-protein diet, as instructed, and every two weeks I dutifully went in to nephrology for the blood and urine tests, creating the time series we needed to write our research paper. I saw the nephrologists every month, and the oncologists every other month. Over the next two months, I had another zero PCR, and my blood and urine protein numbers kept improving. My capacity to walk around improved, too; I lost another five pounds of fluid in my legs and could take stairs and even hike. I was almost feeling normal, and I couldn't help but think that the Rituxan had indeed served a dual purpose, even if it hadn't been proven with clinical trials. "We can't promise this will last," Luis warned, "because some of the few other doctors who tried Rituxan for combating MG found that some patients' MG returned after six to twelve months."

By that time I had been on a half a dozen medical roller coasters, with counts up, counts down, and then back up and back down. I was used to the ups and downs, but I still had trouble accepting with equanimity that I could have a lifetime of treatment roller coasters ahead of me. But I reminded myself that while the numbers oscillated, I was still around and was not suffering acute disease—cancer or kidney. I wasn't really restricted in my activities, so how could I complain? Nevertheless, every now and again the rage, sadness, and consternation that Gary Wynbrandt asked me not to ignore become more than just shadows.

19 | A Successful
Partnership

AT MY NEXT APPOINTMENT in the oncology department in late 2004, I asked Sandra about what we'd do at that point if a PCR test returned a nonzero value. "Rituxan lasts three to six months inside most patients' bodies," she replied, "although it may last longer in yours. We'll have to see what happens when your B cells with CD-20 receptors come back." I agreed that "waiting and seeing" was, once again, our only option.

Sandra surprised us by saying, "We still don't know whether your current zero PCR has any meaning." "What do you mean by that?" I quickly retorted. "It seems obvious I had minimal residual disease and that the Rituxan got rid of it." "No, that's not certain," said Sandra, "because even though the primers used for the PCR are specific to your particular B-cell cancer DNA, other B cells have DNA so close to your cancerous ones that they could fool the primers into thinking you had a very low cancer cell count. There's no telling whether the earlier PCR tests were picking up a false signal or were truly finding cancer cells when they showed low but nonzero values."

Terry and I still had questions about PCR, so Sandra referred us to a research associate in the lab of Dr. James Zehnder, in the pathology department. Dr. Zehnder's lab had performed all my PCR studies. Later, I also found out that the lab was a core facility for conducting research for the bone marrow unit. In the early days of my PCR testing, when I contacted the research associate, she couldn't respond, as it was the lab's policy to provide results only to the requesting physician. But this time, Sandra gave me approval to speak to the research associate, which paved the way for an e-mail conversation between us. The research associate very kindly explained how the PCR test worked and said that based on their experiences, the Zehnder lab thought that the noise level for cancer was a PCR-detected count somewhere between five and fifty cancer cells per microgram of DNA. In an e-mail back to her, I pointed out that the high end of the noise level range was fifty, and I'd had counts of 122 and eighty before. I asked whether 122 could be considered a highly significant signal, given that it was nearly two and a half times greater than fifty. If it was, then maybe the Rituxan maintenance therapy treatments had gotten rid of some real residual cancer. The research associate repeated that we just didn't know how to interpret the low numbers, because there were no large data sets available.

She pointed out that no one knew what a few remaining cancerous cells, as detected by PCR, meant about the possibility of a relapse of mantle cell lymphoma. For other kinds of cancer, some research along these lines had been done. For instance, more PCR testing had been carried out on the blood and tissue samples of chronic myeloid leukemia patients who were in remission, and it was found that people with this kind of cancer can have a low number of cancer cells and not relapse for years. The research associate understood why I was highly interested in being able to interpret my results, and was very sorry that the Zehnder lab simply did not know of data that could help me do so. No such studies were being done then in her department. She suggested that I might want to look for such a study that was going on elsewhere and enroll.

I very much appreciated the research associate's willingness to respond on behalf of the Zehnder lab, but I still don't have any clear interpretation of the difference between noise and signal in the PCR results for my disease. To this day, we are still debating that issue, and my guinea pig status continues.

Winter of My Discontent

In early 2005, my CD-20 B cells reappeared in a blood test—meaning that the Rituxan treatment from six months earlier had finally worn off. Sandra's new oncology Fellow, Natalia Colocci—an M.D. with a Ph.D. in chemistry—took a keen interest in my case, wondering if a PCR test would now show a positive number. If it did, what would it mean? Would it signify that the test was being fooled by the return of benign B cells with CD-20 receptors or that the disappearance of Rituxan from my blood had allowed any remaining cancerous CD-20 B cells to make a comeback—meaning that I had minimal residual disease again?

Natalia e-mailed me in January 2005 telling me that my latest PCR results were in: "Zehnder's lab completed your PCR tests. As you can see, the results are slightly positive [fifty cancer cells per microgram of DNA], but they have been slightly positive before, too. I spoke to Zehnder's associate, and she mentioned that the 'control' yields a value of thirty, and who knows what the error margin on that is." First came the familiar depressive thought: the 500-pound gorilla was stirring again. But at the same time, the very fact that I had a virtual zero cancer count when the CD-20 cells were gone and a small positive number when they came back made us all wonder whether the test was mistaking benign CD-20 cells for malignant ones. I also got to thinking about what it meant that we were now doing PCR tests only on my blood and not on any tissues. The first of my many PCR tests, performed in 2002 on my cancerous lymph node and bone marrow fluid, yielded cancer cell counts of 800,000 and 200,000, respectively. That told me that different tissues can have different cancer cell counts, even if the samples are taken at the same time. Since then, all PCR tests had been performed on my blood—yet a third medium. Even more problematic was the fact that the noise levels that Zehnder's lab reported—PCR results of between five and fifty—were obtained by testing the tonsil tissue of patients who presumably did not have my disease—hence tonsil tissue represented a fourth medium. Could we really compare the PCR numbers for my blood with those for my bone marrow fluid, my lymph nodes, or others' tonsil cells? I suspected not, and I asked Natalia and Sandra to set up a plan to do PCR on at least two different samples—say, my bone marrow fluid and blood—every time I came in for a test. Although I hated the thought of another bone marrow biopsy, the patient from hell is willing to sacrifice his body for science!

Full Partnering

At an appointment in early 2005, Sandra pressed Terry and me on our logic about next steps. I said that I wished that some day, someone, somewhere, would try to clearly define the noise level (or levels, if each tissue has a different one) for PCR so that we could better interpret the test procedure and separate out test error from minimal residual disease. But even in the absence of that information, one thing was certain: When my CD-20 B cells were knocked out by Rituxan—as they were for six months after the four consecutive doses done for maintenance therapy and MG treatment—I had virtually zero cancer counts. "I think it was close to a hard zero," I asserted, "because if I had a lot of cancer hanging around, the PCR would have been able to find it." "I fully agree," Sandra said, "so let me make a proposal." Terry and I were all ears. "Instead of giving you four doses of Rituxan in a month like we did in our first attempt with maintenance therapy, I believe that giving you four doses stretched out over a year will have the same effect, given that Rituxan lasts a long time in your system." I was overjoyed that Sandra was now actually *advocating* maintenance therapy and was pioneering on dosage! "I always wondered if it was overkill giving me four doses in almost immediate succession for maintenance," I agreed. "It would be cheaper to do it this way, and presumably it would have fewer side effects." "But we are pioneering here," Sandra warned, "and there's no telling whether this will be enough." "But if we continue doing PCR regularly," I quickly replied, "we'll know in a matter of a month or two whether our new plan is working. If so, we cheer. If not, we add an extra dose next time and see what the PCR says. I couldn't come up with a better example of Bayesian updating!" I added gleefully. "Good. We agree then," Sandra said. "This may work out very well, and with the PCR test we'll not be taking any dangerous chances."

"Hallelujah!" Terry and I said to each other as we walked out of the hospital, feeling grateful for the fine doctor-patient relationship we had developed with this remarkably open, if megabusy, oncologist. *Soon enough*, I thought, *we should know whether the first low dose of Rituxan led to a negative PCR—molecular remission—or whether we have adjustments to make.* My story may long be a "work in progress," but either way, I hope we'll learn a lot from my stint as guinea pig.

At our most recent meeting as of this writing, Sandra reported that after my maintenance dose of Rituxan in March 2005—the first dose under our new, four times annually plan—a test done on my blood sample taken in May 2005 showed that I had zero CD-20 B cells—and thus a zero cancer count in the PCR was very likely. A week later, Sandra even sent me the expected good news about PCR via e-mail! My next Rituxan treatment will occur in June, followed by PCR in August, Rituxan in September, and so on and so forth, quite possibly for life. I genuinely believe that we can maintain this cycle indefinitely. If it is still working after a few years, I am confident that this treatment or variations that evolve from it will become the norm for treating mantle cell lymphoma patients who have already undergone chemotherapy.

Needless to say, there are no longer any debates with Sandra over whether we should continue the PCR tests; she's as interested in the results as we are. After four years of working together, we have learned firsthand of the benefits of Bayesian updating— not just with the Rituxan for maintenance therapy and treating my MG, but with nearly all aspects of the treatment process. I don't feel anxiety any more when I head in for my appointments; I feel like a partner in a grand experiment that can save my life and just maybe help many others too. That is what science—medicine included—is supposed to be about.

The Continuing Saga

On May 3, 2005, I was interviewed in the *New York Times* by Claudia Dreifus about my treatments and about this book. It set off a battle among oncologists that I think is very healthy. Progressives, like Sandra Horning and Alessandro Gianni, are pitted against traditionalists, who still insist that without clinical trials data, innovative treatments like our four Rituxan per year maintenance therapy are foolish and perhaps dangerous. The conservatives cite long-term data showing that for mantle cell lymphoma patients, standard CHOP chemotherapy produces outcomes statistically similar to CHOP plus Rituxan—that is, many patients lost remission after about five years. The conservatives treat this as proof that Rituxan is not effective in treating mantle cell lymphoma. However, I believe their logic is flawed; one needs only to consider the dynamics of exponential population growth to understand how.

Imagine that before treatment, two acutely ill patients each had, say, 100 billion cancer cells threatening their lives. Suppose that one patient received CHOP, which reduced his cancer cell count to 100,000. Let's assume that patient 2 received CHOP plus Rituxan. Considerable data show that in the short term, Rituxan *does* reduce cancer cell counts, so with CHOP plus Rituxan, the patient might end up with something like 1,000 remaining cancer cells. Then, for the next several years, some combination of the patients' own immunities and slow growth of the residual cancer cells delays the exponential explosion of cancer for, say, five years. Then exponential growth takes over in both patients. Given the nature of exponential growth, it wouldn't matter whether the cancer count started at 10, 100, 10,000, or 100,000 cells, since eventually the results of the exponential growth would be the same. So are the conservatives right that Rituxan is ineffective in the long term for mantle cell lymphoma? Absolutely not. The flaw in their logic is that they are not considering Rituxan for use as maintenance therapy. One can't assume that Rituxan is ineffective as maintenance therapy by looking at long-term data in which no maintenance therapy was performed! My case should prove that it *is* effective over time, as I didn't do maintenance therapy until three years after transplant and the Rituxan immediately achieved molecular remission for me.

This can be viewed as a classic predator-prey situation, and an ecological analogy I can use to describe it is one of rabbits and foxes. Cancer cells are akin to rabbits; Rituxan and T cells are like two species of foxes. A person's cancer most likely begins when his or her T cell foxes are weak, which allows the rabbit population—the cancer cells—to grow exponentially. Then, during treatment, a patient's own foxes are aided by new foxes in the form of chemotherapy drugs and perhaps radiation. This reduces the rabbit population to a very low level, which is why after treatment, a patient may be in remission for many years. His or her own foxes may be able to keep the rabbit population under control. But eventually the balance may tip, and the rabbits may begin to grow exponentially again. At that point, it doesn't matter whether the rabbit population starts at 10 or 1,000 (which may be the difference between CHOP and CHOP plus Rituxan); exponential growth is exponential growth. Whatever the initial number of posttreatment rabbits, the results of such rapid multiplication will be the same once an exponential growth phase occurs. The goal is to keep the rabbits from reaching carrying capacity, at which point the patient would be dead. To achieve this, maintenance therapy with Rituxan could be performed, so that the T cell foxes have some powerful backup. Together, the Rituxan and T cells can hopefully keep the cancer under control well past the five-year point.

While this may sound like another wacky theory from the patient from hell, Dr. Gianni recently confirmed that we may not be too far off. After reading the manuscript for this book, Dr. Gianni sent an e-mail updating me on the test group of patients reported on in his paper in *Blood* (discussed in chapter 17). All the patients in his test group are still alive and cancer free. Two of the patients had positive PCRs after a couple of years, and after treatment with Rituxan, both reachieved molecular remission—just like I have three years out.

Of course, it will be difficult to "prove it" statistically or to convince conservative doctors of the merit of Rituxan for maintenance therapy until actual Rituxan maintenance clinical trials data are available—but perhaps the good process knowledge applied by Drs. Horning and Gianni, combined with preliminary evidence, including my own, will convince more medical practitioners to adopt individualization as a standard operating procedure and, in the case of B-cell lymphomas, engage in more extensive clinical trials using Rituxan as maintenance therapy after conventional high-dose initial treatments. Meanwhile, before those data eventually dribble in, I hope my fellow patients will insist that these options be seriously considered and openly discussed among them, their physicians, and their advocates.

CHAPTER

20 | You and Your Docs:

Allies, Not Adversaries

SINCE UNDERGOING TREATMENT for my cancer, I have received numerous e-mails, phone calls, and letters from personal friends, colleagues, and others who have been diagnosed with cancer, asking for my advice. Although I am not a medical doctor and am not in a position to give medical guidance to anyone—and in fact it would be quackery for me to do so—I certainly have enough experience to advise people about what types of questions they could ask their doctors. I have stressed over and over and over again in long phone calls and e-mail exchanges with these genuinely worried people, with diseases of various sorts and in various stages, the absolutely essential nature of pressing for individualized diagnostics and of assuring that they're not being treated as "mythical average patients."

My goal in these interactions—and in this book—is to encourage patient-physician interaction, cooperation, and a broadening of the way treatments are designed. No one should look for medical advice in this book—get that from your doctors and your advocate. (Several places to begin are given in the Web site guide at the end of the book.) However, the applications of decision analysis to problems marked with great uncertainties—an essential core of my life's work—is often underrepresented in the practice of medicine. I am hoping that this book helps nudge medical schools and hospitals not only to require more extensive decision-analysis training for all students, but also to emphasize the *practical* application of decision analysis. When medical students begin doing clinical rotations, and later residencies, that would seem a good time to teach them how and when to apply decision analysis. This kind of learning-by-doing would cement the theoretical-level decision analysis taught in medical school by providing a transition to real-life situations. For current practitioners far past residency, seminars or refresher courses that emphasize applications of decision-analysis techniques would seem very prudent.

Fighting Your Own Battle

You may be asking yourself, "How can I be the 'patient from hell'?" You may have enjoyed some of my stories but feel that it would be impossible for you to replicate my actions, especially if it means wrestling face-to-face with the often hierarchical medical profession and bureaucratic insurance companies or HMOs. This can be particularly difficult if you are gravely ill or feel insufficiently informed to argue cogently with doctors locked into certain protocols and hospitals or insurance companies clinging to self-interested business practices.

If this is you, do not despair. It's very important to understand that I did not write this book to convince people that the only course of action in pursuing optimum treatment for life-threatening medical conditions is to act just like I did, questioning and confronting "the system" every other step of the way. I think that might work for some of you, and certainly I hope you will all take away the message that the better informed you are, the better your outcome will be, at least if you learn to decide how to take risks more appropriately for yourself. Just being aware of how hospitals and the doctors within them operate should give you some leverage and understanding in dealing with your disease and your treatment team.

But remember, there is an alternative to becoming another patient from hell: Get an advocate. You don't need a Ph.D. or an M.D. to become your own advocate or to have a patient advocate working for you. You and your advocate just need to remember the three questions of scientific literacy: 1) What can happen? 2) What are the odds of it happening? And, most important when talking with your medical professionals: 3) How do you know and how can you verify the answers to the first two questions? Not only do you need to know your doctors' estimates of the likelihoods of various events related to your health, but *you need to know how confident they are in their estimates of these likelihoods.* If clinical trials data for your disease are scarce, as is often the case, or if the clinical trials show a wide spectrum of outcomes across a diverse patient population, then you must accept that your doctors cannot truly be confident in their predictions about your particular case, especially if you are very different from the average patient. You, a family member, or a professional advocate can ask these questions and, with your doctors, formulate a plan for getting the most appropriate treatment for *your specific, individual needs.*

Back in the Game

Maybe retired doctors would make excellent patient advocates. This would be akin to a senior professor becoming a professor emeritus who keeps her office and still teaches her favorite class but can skip the tedium of faculty meetings, dean's pronouncements, and so on. Becoming patient advocates would permit retired doctors to stay in the game they know so well without having to attend department meetings or be on call late nights, weekends, or for emergencies. This could prove to be the best of both worlds for them. It would be beneficial to patients, too, since retired doctors working as advocates would likely be credible to practicing docs. Who will pay for such services is still a subject of debate, with proponents suggesting that patient advocacy is a legitimate and effective health care expense that should be covered by insurance, while others, I suspect, consider it an unnecessary luxury or even a time-consuming interference with medicine-as-usual. While my sympathies lie with the proponents, fair rules on who pays for patient advocates will likely require further public debate—and perhaps legislation.

Some friends and colleagues of mine have balked at my retired-doc-as-patient-advocate idea, suggesting that retired doctors may be very set in their ways and unwilling to modernize. They may not embrace—or even understand—the principles of Bayesian updating and decision analysis. However, as I argued in the preface, retired doctors *do* have a wealth of medical information, and they are more likely than an overly busy practicing doc to have the time to brush up on decision analysis through a refresher course, informational reading, or Web sources—once they exist.

Decision Analysis and the Precautionary Principle

Being an advocate for yourself or someone else can be stressful, and it often involves dealing with a doctor who is so busy that the extra time you demand will undoubtedly be burdensome. I'm sure at times Sandra Horning tired of Terry's and my constant questions and challenges, and I know that she was busy to the point of exhaustion. I'm sure that overcommitted doctors are often tempted to follow a battlefield triage approach, treating every patient according to the protocol and avoiding the extra hours it would take to fashion individualizations. I am grateful that Sandra took the time to pursue individualization in my case. Despite the extra time it took, I think she came to enjoy and value our interactions. Otherwise, she wouldn't have convinced her colleagues to modify protocols for me, nor would she have gone on to do the same for other patients. I greatly value her flexibility in our discussions, though we still debate the pros and cons of various decision rules. However, I now believe that Sandra and quite a few other docs agree more with the decision-analysis style Terry and I negotiated than I originally thought. I think, too, that over time, many more scientists will accept applications of the precautionary principle, whether it is in relation to stemming climate change or cancer, especially when the costs of precautionary actions are low and the relative potential benefits high.

It's the System, Not the Doctor

Although some doctors may largely agree with me about individualizing testing and treatments, many are embedded in a system that doesn't always promote practices based on decision analysis or the precautionary principle. It is therefore one of my hoped-for objectives that this book will not only encourage patients to press their doctors to perform individualized diagnostics—and when appropriate, change protocols—but also convince frustrated doctors to press hospitals, HMOs, and the government to change the system so that individualization and patient advocacy become the rule, not the exception. I am optimistic that most doctors reading this book will not think of me as hostile to them, but grateful for their dedication, for their research, and for saving my life. I hope that more doctors will apply their decision-analysis skills and consider whether allowing accountant-determined "costs" to dictate medical protocols is really "best practice," even if it means confronting the bureaucracies within which they operate. I'm calling on all who agree that the system needs major reforming to muster their courage and challenge it. Patients and advocates can do only so much. We can push for changes at the individual level, but it is up to health professionals to implement systemwide changes in their domain. I would no more expect to broker changes in medical institutions than to anticipate doctors forcing action in climate change decision making. But either can report what we see and ask insiders to act.

In the immediate future, I suggest that medical institutions at least strive for partial individualization. For example, they might come up with diagnostic testing that separates patients into three categories. If the diagnostics show that the patient has a relatively mild case of a particular disease, the patient would be placed in the first category, which would correspond to lower-intensity treatments. If the diagnostics revealed that the patient's disease was of average severity, he or she would be placed in the second category, which would correspond to the standard protocol. If the patient was found to have a worse-than-average case, he or she would be placed in the third category and would receive treatments more aggressive than the protocol used with the average patients. Of course, given the lack of data available for such partitioning, it is essential that frequent and powerful individualized diagnostic tests be performed to indicate whether the plan is working.

For most cancer patients in major institutions, their cancer is typed and staged, and the severity of their disease is determined. But does this translate to differentiated treatments according to the individualized diagnostics? I suspect that the answer is sometimes yes, sometimes no. In the future, I hope the answer is a consistent yes and that as treatment progresses, it is coupled with individualized testing. In addition, such a system can be adhered to even by doctors who aren't current on medical breakthroughs and recent literature, particularly if authoritative Web sites were available that detailed the kinds of individualized tests to perform and treatments to match the results.

Did Individualization Really Help Me?

You may be wondering why I am advocating for these changes, given that I still don't know if I've seen the last of my cancer. Did all my pushing for individualization really make any difference? In truth, there were times in writing this book when I thought, *You still may get back acute cancer, so who are you to give advice to other people about getting involved in stressful dialogues when you may not be in remission that long yourself?* I will never know for certain what would have happened if Terry and I had not intervened and Sandra had not responded so positively. I can't say how my health would be today had I not surreptitiously scheduled two additional blood tests and gotten Neupogen, not had PCR, not lobbied for the Isolex 300i blood-purging machine, not pressed my doctors into giving me whole-body radiation even though I was one year past the age limit specified by the protocol, not been reinforced by Dr. Gianni's strong opinion on maintenance therapy, and not finally gotten Rituxan for my MG and for maintenance therapy, which I believe is responsible for reducing my cancer cell count—at least so far—to zero, or what we hope is a negligible number. How would my story read in the absence of these individualizations? We cannot yet know which aspects of my individualized treatment were more and less effective (as that will require frequency data), but overall, I suspect my story would be worse without it. Perhaps I would have ended up with the same PCR range of 20–120 cancer cells per microgram of DNA if my treatment had followed a standard protocol, but I might also have ended up with 200,000 and been back where I started: in the hospital undergoing another very costly, life-threatening, organ-damaging set of treatments, with an even bleaker outlook, at high expense to me, the hospital, and the insurance company.

Despite the unknowns, I'd be willing to bet that if a bunch of informed patients acted as their own advocates or appointed advocates to work for them, and a bunch of others didn't, the group that took the advocacy approach would have the better outcomes. This would be an excellent topic of study for a public health researcher. Until such a study exists, I can only extrapolate the results of my personal experiences with cancer to mean that strong patient-doctor partnerships are more effective than the more traditional passive-patient alternatives. So far, so good for me, but real data on a large patient population would be better.

Many important things in life—from treating cancer to acting on the potential risks posed by climate change—are a gamble and are subjects for which we don't have enough data to be completely certain about possible outcomes and their likelihoods. Like many other big problems, cancer and climate change are marked by deep uncertainties, lack adequate data, are plagued by ideological adherence to methods and policies that don't necessarily constitute "best practice," and are embedded in systems that consider private costs ahead of social costs and hierarchies that often elevate the opinions of professionals on the basis of status rather than process knowledge, data, and experience. The best we can do in dealing with these problems is to learn to understand the processes involved, work to minimize risks, and then deal with what risks remain in a way that best matches our value systems.

As I mentioned in chapter 10 (and alluded to in the preface) I often think of life as a roulette wheel containing both happy and nasty outcomes. No matter what we do, sometimes the roulette wheel presents us with lousy results. While we can't always prevent undesirable events from occurring, I do think there is always something we can do to narrow the width of the slots that represent poor consequences and widen those that imply good outcomes. In the case of cancer, that "something" is learning more about what can happen, what the odds are, and how we can improve our chances. Don't take a fatalistic approach when dealing with your diagnosis; get an advocate, get involved with your treatment, and work with your doctors to tailor an individualized solution if doing so seems better for your case than following a standard protocol to the letter.

The medical establishment can also help to narrow the nasty slots on each of our roulette wheels. Scientific literacy, openness, full cost accounting (not just a focus on private costs), caring about the future and those who are or will be affected by their decisions, and individualizing treatments would be my prescription for hospitals, insurance companies, HMOs, legislators, and doctors who want to improve patients' odds and to find the most cost-effective solutions to uncertainty-ridden problems, especially in the treatment of rare diseases.

Becoming a "patient from hell" or a proactive patient of any sort may well delay your trip to the next world. Regardless of whether you believe in such things, stay alive and make a difference! For many of us, our responsibility to ourselves and to posterity is what keeps us going. I intend to keep battling, both on cancer treatment and on climate change policy, as long as I'm in this life and these problems still exist. I guess that means I'll be pretty busy for the foreseeable future. Thanks to my treatment team, I actually have a foreseeable future.

A Caregiver's Journey

Terry L. Root

Many people say that dealing with cancer is like riding a roller coaster. But it is not that tame. It's more like riding a roller coaster blindfolded—or, rather, like being blindfolded and forced onto and off of different rides, some terrifying, some soothing. You never know what the next ride will be, what to expect, or when to expect it. At times life is a joy because of a newfound realization of the importance of being together. Most of the time, however, all you can do is brace yourself as your world seems to drop out from under you.

When Steve found the lump under his arm, neither of us thought much about it. We were quite vigilant about the possibility of my getting cancer, because of my extensive family history of breast cancer; but Steve's family history of cancer is next to nil. (His mother contracted lung cancer at age eighty, but it almost certainly was caused by her decades of heavy smoking.) As the months passed and the lump persisted, though, we became more and more concerned about it. On the day of Steve's first biopsy, we knew there was trouble when the doctors discovered that there were more lumps than the one we knew about. At that very moment I took on a new role in life—supporter and caregiver to the man who is my best friend and whom I love more than words can express.

My new role began in earnest when we got the results of the biopsy. As Steve recounted in his story, he got the news in the Baltimore airport. I had already boarded our plane and was settling in for a cross-country flight. Then Steve arrived. One glance told me our lives had just taken a horrible turn. He was pale, his every muscle was tense, and when he looked into my eyes, I could see his fear, which made our love for each other even more meaningful. After getting his luggage stored and buckling up in the seat next to mine, Steve explained that his doctor just told him he had non-Hodgkin's lymphoma but that the particular type was not known yet. At that point the type did not matter. What mattered was being together. My caregiving role began in the form of quiet, loving support. I took Steve's hands in mine and said very calmly, "We can fight this together. You are strong and we are a formidable pair. We can do this together."

During what seemed to be the longest flight in the history of aviation, we held on to each other for dear life. I followed Steve's lead: If he wanted to talk, I'd listen and respond. If he sat quietly, I just held him. Somewhere along the way, I did cry, both with Steve and alone.

The next day, I bought a large spiral notebook with five sections: one for notes taken when talking with doctors; one for recording medications, doses, and dates given; one for questions Steve or I thought about between doctor visits; one for notes taken from the Internet and other sources; and one for anything else that needed to be recorded. That same day, armed with my notebook and pen, I walked hand-in-hand with Steve into Oncology Day Care.

Waiting in an exam room for your first oncology visit is pure torture. I came prepared with plenty of stories, questions, and information to use to help distract Steve while we waited, but it wasn't very effective. Finally, the oncology Fellow knocked and entered. I whipped out my notebook and pen.

As the Fellow spoke, I began writing notes at high speed; I didn't want to miss a thing. I kept wishing I'd brought a tape recorder. I suspended my emotions as well as I could in order to get down all the information coming from the Fellow and later from the oncologist, Sandra Horning. Still, there were two moments when my emotions just came flying out unchecked and uncontrollable. The first was when we were told that Steve had mantle cell lymphoma. The actual diagnosis meant nothing to us at the time, but the way the Fellow said, "You have mantle cell lymphoma" sent an ice pick through my heart. His tone said that this was not one of the "easy-to-fight" lymphomas.

The second time my emotions erupted was when Sandra started explaining the treatment. During that first meeting, I repeated a plea over and over again in my head: "Please don't recommend a bone marrow transplant as part of his treatment!" While on the faculty at the University of Michigan, I had a student in one of my classes who underwent two such transplants. We talked about his experiences, because I sensed that he wanted someone who cared to talk about those tough times in his life. He explained how physically and emotionally demanding the transplants were for him, but he was glad to have done them because the procedures had saved his life, making it possible for him to return to school and a normal life.

My mental pleas did no good whatsoever. My hopes were shattered when Sandra said that Steve would need an autologous stem cell replacement—a bone marrow transplant. Another ice pick pierced my heart.

After both of these pronouncements, I needed a moment to think and to compose myself, but the information kept flowing. My job as note taker didn't allow me the luxury of focusing on my feelings.

I must have done a good job of suspending my emotions because I took copious notes. Looking back on that appointment, I only remember hearing the Fellow give us Steve's diagnosis and Sandra Horning's initial words about treatments. But somehow I managed to take pages and pages of notes, full of explicit details about everything that occurred during the meeting.

Next we learned that Steve needed to have a bone marrow biopsy, right then and there. The rudimentary aspects of what was to be done were explained to us, but neither of us was prepared for this truly scary and painful procedure. Steve was stretched out on the examining table, lying on his stomach, and I stood by his side holding his hand. Steve was facing me, but I was facing the Fellow and watching him assemble the instruments. I remember thinking, *It looks as though the mental torture Steve just endured is going to be matched by the physical torture to be inflicted by those instruments.* I was right. He was given lidocaine at the location of the puncture, but that was not sufficient to stop the pain.

When the instrument punched through Steve's bone with a crunch, I felt a viselike grip on my hand. Simultaneously, I became very light-headed, which had never happened to me before. Being the caregiver and not the care receiver, I told myself I could not faint. I had to find some way to get my head closer to the floor while still providing Steve with much-needed comfort. I squatted so that I could look directly into Steve's eyes, all the while keeping up a conversation that I hoped was helping to distract us both from the torture. The fright in Steve's eyes drove away all my light-headedness in a second—and the squatting certainly helped some too.

Sandra had told us not to look up mantle cell lymphoma on the Web, because under the old protocols—the ones we'd primarily find on the Web—the average life expectancy was two to three years. Under the new protocol of CHOP plus Rituxan, all of Sandra's patients were still alive after four years. As we walked to the car after that first meeting, Steve and I agreed that he would not use the Web to learn about his lymphoma. I was the designated Web searcher and would pass on needed information to him. This rule turned out to be a good one because it prevented Steve from undergoing a lot of unneeded anxiety. At the same time, however, my role as information filter caused me to endure some lonely suffering, which at times was quite difficult. Thank heavens for friends and the caregivers support group!

Our friends and families became my anchors. All those in my situation will find help in their own way, but let me give you three examples that were very important to me. First, our longtime friend and colleague at Stanford, Paul Ehrlich, came to the hospital every day to visit Steve in the clean room and see how we were doing. This required that he scrub his hands and forearms for three minutes straight and then put on a gown and a mask. Before he left each day, Paul was always sure to give me a big hug and to remind me that I needed to take care of myself. After each of his visits, Paul e-mailed a progress report on Steve to a group of our mutual friends, who in turn forwarded the e-mail to other friends of ours. In this way, a large network of people was able to keep track of Steve's progress without my lifting a finger.

Perhaps my greatest anchor was my brother, Bryan, who is as busy or busier than the rest of us, because he is the owner of a small high-tech company. When Steve was diagnosed with mantle cell lymphoma, Bryan told me that if I needed him at any time he would get on a plane and be there. I did not think I would take him up on his offer, but when Steve was at his worst—needing a lot of morphine and an antifungal drug to prevent infection—I called Bryan. He arrived early the next day. He saw how tired I was and made me promise to call him if I was not going to be able to get home from the hospital by 2:00 a.m. Between midnight and 1:00, Steve started shaking uncontrollably because of a reaction to his antifungal medication. The nurses stopped the drip feed of medication, and after a while the shaking stopped. Once Steve fell asleep, I called Bryan. The next thing I knew, he was outside Steve's room scrubbing and donning a gown and mask. Bryan told me to go home and sleep, and he promised to stay with Steve until

I came back the next morning. I was so very touched by my brother's love and caring that I cried myself to sleep that night.

My other friends also provided an endless stream of love and support. Before Steve went into the hospital, there were times when he needed a lot of my attention. My wonderful friends Liz Hadley and Angela Riccelli knew that these were tough times for me and that I had little time to cook. On the days that were particularly difficult, one or the other of them always seemed to show up near dinnertime with an entire home-cooked meal ready to eat. They gave me not only nutritious and wonderfully delicious meals, but also the caregiving that I needed to be a strong caregiver for Steve.

Then the day arrived for Steve to check into the hospital. That first day was difficult; we had to get used to Steve's not only being in the hospital, but being in the clean room. I stayed at the hospital quite late—later than I'd planned, because I had locked my keys in the car, which shows how preoccupied I was that morning. When I finally arrived home in Paul Ehrlich's "taxi," waiting for me on the porch was a beautiful flower arrangement from two friends, Gretchen Daily and Gideon Yoffe. I put the flowers in our bedroom, where I would see them first thing in the morning and last thing at night. I am very lucky to have such caring and supportive friends and family. My job would have been almost impossible without such an outpouring of love.

Like many others, I also got a lot of help from the hospital-arranged caregivers support group. The meetings, attended mostly by spouses of stem-cell-replacement patients, provided a very welcome framework that allowed me to reveal my anxiety, anger, joy, exhaustion, and ever-present fear. At the first meeting I attended, the other caregivers and I shared some laughs and many tears. I quickly developed a mutual trust with those present, some of whom became close friends. For most if not all of us, the probability that any of our spouses would die was much, much higher than it had ever been before. We were all doing everything we could to wrestle that probability down as low as possible, but life and death were now so closely intertwined that we had to accept a new reality.

As Steve explains in this book, he is proud of the fact that he was able to undertake many of his normal day-to-day tasks throughout most of his treatment. He is proud of the fact that he was able to conduct as much business from his hospital bed as he did. Part of my "job," however, was to try to get him to rest enough to allow his body to heal. For any caregiver, this task can be quite challenging. Additionally, I was concerned that his being confined in the hospital would drive him crazy, especially because Steve is such a "people person." Being the caregiver, I felt it was my job to distract him so that his feelings of confinement were minimal. With this in mind, I hatched four plans. The first was to bring to the hospital all the pictures we had ever taken, sort them into trips or years, and put them into photo albums. The doctors and nurses could not believe the number of pictures I brought in, but I had to be armed with fun memories to help Steve (and me) get through what turned out to be some pretty tough times. When Steve was sleeping, I would quietly put photos in the albums. When he was awake, we would look at pictures and talk about all the memories that surfaced.

My second plan was to reinforce Steve's sense of the many people who truly care about him. To do this I got a huge piece of construction paper and wrote in big letters, "STEVE, YOU ARE IN OUR THOUGHTS!" I put it up on the wall of the clean room so Steve could see it from his bed. Then when someone would call, come by, send an e-mail or card, or pass along their good wishes via another friend, I wrote their name on the sign. By the end of his stay, the sign was completely covered with names. It really helped to raise both Steve's and my spirits.

The third plan gave us a focus several years beyond the hospital and cancer. Together, we began organizing a large scientific symposium to be held in conjunction with Steve's sixtieth birthday. Steve is a world-renowned scientist who has had a lot of influence on many scientists, policymakers, business people, and the general public. His fifty-seventh birthday came just a couple of weeks after he got out of the hospital. Thinking about a big event that would take place three years in the future gave us something fun and important to look forward to. We enjoyed putting together a preliminary agenda for the symposium and coming up with a guest list. I must admit that I was concerned about the possibility of having a memorial symposium. Thankfully, Steve was there to attend the three-day symposium, which was held in February 2005. It was a wonderful success and a fabulous celebration of Steve's sixty years. All the speakers attested to Steve's important influence in their lives and on their careers—a legacy that will endure through time. One of the most poignant comments was the private confession from a friend who is a journalist that he was thrilled to have been deprived of writing an obituary for Steve. Steve joked that he was flattered to learn that such a well-known journalist was slated to pen that document but that he intended to continue to deprive him of the need to do so.

The fourth plan was one designed simply to help us get through one day at a time. This involved watching reruns of the television show *Northern Exposure*. We love that show. Being from New York City, Steve gets a kick out of the different issues that Joel Fleischman, a doctor originally from New York City, has to contend with the small town in Alaska where he works. Before I left for the hospital each day, I set the VCR to record that day's rerun, and I would take the previous day's recording to the hospital. Around 10:00 each night, I would wheel the TV/VCR into Steve's room so we could watch the previous day's recordings. I would sit next to Steve, holding his hand, and we would both be whisked from Stanford Hospital to Cicely, Alaska, for an hour.

Even when he was at his lowest point—when the radiation damage and the effects of having no stem cells were at their worst—Steve remembered my birthday and even managed to arrange a surprise party. Every day, I got to the hospital no later than 9:00 a.m. and never left before 11:00 p.m. I was reluctant to change that schedule, even on my birthday, but Steve finally convinced me to leave the hospital early to go to dinner with Angela Riccelli and her husband, Larry Goulder. I drove straight from the hospital to their house, and we walked to a nearby restaurant. I was so preoccupied that it was not until I was literally standing behind my chair that I realized that there were already people sitting at the table. All of them were close friends who wanted to help me celebrate my birthday. I was overwhelmed. The love that those friends and others have for both Steve and me continue to make our coping with cancer bearable.

This cancer adventure has pushed Steve and me to physical and emotional extremes, both positive and negative. My journey, like those of many spouses and caregivers, started with numbness and evolved into a protecting, supporting, and information-gathering state. From there, I found myself feeling angry because if Steve were to die, I was the one who would be left without the person who means the most to me in my life. Finally, after a while, I was able to step back and be grateful for the challenges we went through because they brought us to a new level of love—one where we appreciate every moment we have, both together and alone.

So now I need to revise the first paragraph of this afterword. Dealing with cancer is indeed like being blindfolded and put on different rides, but now I know that these rides have safety mechanisms. They are the many people standing close by waiting to provide whatever is needed to help buffer the difficult times and celebrate the pleasures with us as we travel a journey we never wanted to take.

Preface: I'm Just a Patient—Doesn't the Doctor Know Best?

1. Murdock, R., and D. Fisher, 2000: *Patient Number One: A True Story of How One CEO Took on Cancer and Big Business in the Fight of His Life* (New York: Crown Publishers).

2. Armstrong, L., and S. Jenkins, 2000: *It's Not About the Bike: My Journey Back to Life* (New York: Putnam Publishing Group).

Chapter 1: "But Doctor, It Takes Three Tests to Find the Bottom"

1. In fact, I "gamed the system" once again and scheduled a blood test about seven days before my second round of chemo and was shocked to see that my white blood count was over 7,000—higher than normal for me despite the chemo! It signaled that the Neupogen was working. In addition, when I took the normally scheduled blood test fourteen days after the second chemo, my white count was only suppressed to about 3,500, a far cry from the 500 count I had after the first round of chemo. I never added any blood tests again after that and went along with the doctors' single-nadir measurement fourteen days after chemo. I also went to work daily, even during my nadir weeks, which eliminated the whopping cost to me, to Stanford, and to society of a lost work week.

Chapter 2: This Better Not Be Serious—I've Got a Plane to Catch

1. Phlebitis is an inflammation of a vein, commonly associated with clot formation and partial or complete obstruction of the flow of blood in the vessel.

2. These problems are examples of what sociologists Silvio Funtowicz and Jerome Ravetz call "postnormal science." In what Thomas Kuhn described as "normal science," we scientists go to our labs and we make our usual measurements, calculate our usual statistics, build our usual models, and proceed on a particular well-established paradigm. Postnormal science, on the other hand, acknowledges that while we're doing our normal science, some groups want or need to know the answers well before normal science has resolved the deep inherent uncertainties surrounding the problem at hand. Such groups have a stake in the outcome and want some way of dealing with the vast array of uncertainties—which, by the way, are not all equal in the degree of confidence they carry. Compared with applied science and professional consultancy, postnormal science carries both higher decision stakes and higher systems uncertainty.

I explain it in more detail on my climate change Web site: http://stephenschneider. stanford.edu/Climate/Climate_Policy/CliPolFrameset.html.

3. For additional information on Bayesian updating, see Charness, G., and D. Levin, 2003: "Bayesian Updating vs. Reinforcement and Affect: A Laboratory Study," Ohio State University working paper (http://economics.sbs.ohio-state.edu/levin/wpapers/ charness_levin.pdf). The classical work in the context of decision analysis is Morgan, M. G., and M. Henrion, 1990: *Uncertainty: A Guide to Dealing with Uncertainty in Quantitative Risk and Policy Analysis.* Cambridge, England: Cambridge University Press. However, it is written for professionals and has a high entry bar in terms of mathematical prerequisites. Richard Berk, of the University of California, Los Angeles, also explains the concepts of Bayesian updating simply and qualitatively. See Berk, R., 1996: "Bayesian Approaches to Characterizing Uncertainty," presentation in Session II (Characterizing and Communicating Scientific Uncertainty) at Aspen Global Change Institute meeting, 31 July—8 August (http://www.agci.org/publications/ eoc96/AGCIEOC96SSSII/AGCIEOC96BerkSSSII.html).

4. Article 2 of the United Nations Framework Convention on Climate Change states: "The ultimate objective of this Convention and any related legal instruments that the Conference of the Parties may adopt is to achieve, in accordance with the relevant provisions of the Convention, stabilization of greenhouse gas concentrations in the atmosphere at a level that would prevent dangerous anthropogenic interference with the climate system." The Framework Convention on Climate Change further suggests that "such a level should be achieved within a time frame sufficient to allow ecosystems to adapt naturally to climate change, to ensure that food production is not threatened and to enable economic development to proceed in a sustainable manner."

5. This statement appeared in Working Group II's Summary for Policymakers, part of the IPCC Third Assessment Report.

Chapter 3: Whew! The Tests Are Negative, and I've Got a Plane to Catch

1. The Kyoto Protocol is the voluntary (and only!) international agreement on greenhouse gas abatement. It was drawn up in Kyoto, Japan, in 1997 by the Conference of the Parties to United Nations Framework Convention on Climate Change. Its goal is for developed countries to reduce greenhouse gas emissions by an average of 5.2 percent below 1990 levels by 2012 through abatement, which can be in the form of either direct emissions rules—called "command and control regulations"—or market mechanisms such as carbon taxes or trading regimes in which bigger polluters would pay lesser polluters for emissions rights, creating a market for carbon emissions. (Economic theory and much empirical evidence show that market mechanisms are usually the much cheaper way to achieve an emissions target.) Developed countries would be required to begin reducing emissions in 2008. Developing nations are not committed to any emissions reductions in the first round but will be under pressure to adhere to targets in later rounds if the protocol is to be effective over time. In order for the protocol to go into effect, countries that were responsible for at least 55 percent of 1990 greenhouse gas emissions must sign it. Because countries such as the United States and Australia are resisting becoming signatories, the protocol did not go into effect until October 2004, after Russia ratified it, only after the European Union promised it would fight for Russia's entry into the World Trade Organization.

2. Coal industry data from Australia's Department of Industry, Tourism, and Resources (http://www.industry.gov.au/coal) and from Gladstone Centre for Clean Coal (http://gc3.cqu.edu.au/modern-world/index.php).

3. Tom Lovejoy is president of the Heinz Center for Science, Economics, and the Environment, chief biodiversity adviser to the World Bank, and senior adviser to the president of the UN Foundation. He is credited with coining the term "biological diversity" and pioneered the idea of "debt for nature swaps." To solve the two seemingly intractable problems of loss of nature and financial debt in developing countries, he proposes that richer donor nations forgive a portion of the debt accrued by developing countries in exchange for the latter's protecting their threatened forests, wetlands, and other natural resources.

Chapter 4: Taking My Lumps: Biopsy Blues

1. Dr. Harry Oberhelman, a general surgeon, retired in October 2002, after forty-two years of service at the Stanford Medical Center.

2. The difference between B-cell and T-cell cancer is the type of cell infected with cancer (B cells versus T cells). B cells, also called B lymphocytes, are white blood cells that make antibodies and are an important part of the immune system. B cells come from bone marrow. T cells are a specific type of white blood cell that attacks virus-infected cells, foreign cells, and cancer cells. T cells also produce a number of substances that regulate the immune response.

3. Dr. Ronald Levy is a professor of oncology at Stanford University Medical Center. His research focuses on the study of malignant lymphoma and tumors of the immune system using the tools of immunology and molecular biology to develop a better understanding of the initiation and progression of the malignant process.

4. Louis Pitelka is a professor at the University System of Maryland and director of the Appalachian Laboratory, an environmental research facility of the University of Maryland Center for Environmental Science.

5. Chronic lymphocytic leukemia (CLL) is the most common type of leukemia contracted by adults; about 7,000 new cases are diagnosed each year in the United States. A telltale sign of the cancer is the production of abnormal white blood cells that survive for an uncharacteristically long time. The abnormal white cells accumulate slowly, eventually crowding out healthy white cells, platelets, and red blood cells. There is no cure yet for CLL, and treatment usually does not begin until the patient exhibits symptoms. Patients are expected to live, on average, for about ten years after contracting the disease, but with newer treatments that number is increasing. Information obtained from http://www.chronic-leukemia-and-symptoms.com/html/chronic-lymphocytic-leukemia.php3.

6. A computed tomography (CT) scan provides X-ray images created by a computerized synthesis of X-ray data from many different angles in one plane or cross-section at a time. Typically images are taken of multiple planes a few millimeters apart. Computers can also generate 3-D images of an anatomic structure using two-dimensional X-ray pictures, one slice at a time.

7. In a positron emission tomography (PET) scan, a solution containing a small dose of a positron-emitting radionuclide combined with a sugar is injected into the patient. A PET scanner then rotates around the patient's head and progresses down the body, detecting the positron emissions given off by the radionuclide. The computer produces a color-coded picture based on the measurements of glucose used in different regions. Because malignant tumors usually grow very quickly compared with normal, healthy tissue, tumor cells will consume more sugar and will appear in a different color or shade on the image.

8. Schmidt, K., and E. Ernst, 2004: "Assessing websites on alternative and complementary information for cancer," *Annals of Oncology* 15: 733–742.

Chapter 5: "Once Per Lethal Disease": Coping with Chemo

1. A monoclonal antibody is a laboratory-produced protein that can find particular kinds of cells (B cells in my case), including cancerous ones, wherever they are in the body and attach itself to them. Different types of monoclonal antibodies recognize different proteins on different types of cells. They can be used alone or as messengers for carrying drugs, toxins, or radioactive material to cells. Mature B cells have CD-20 receptor sites.

2. An important concept in the evolution of cancer therapy was to combine agents with different mechanisms of action and nonoverlapping toxicity. Combining Rituxan with chemo was a perfect application of this concept, since Rituxan killed B cells differently than chemo and didn't possess the usual dangers of chemotherapy.

3. In solid (rather than IV liquid) form, Kytril, a highly effective antinausea medicine, costs $50 a pill. As a result, a patient cannot get a prescription for more than three pills at a time; insurance companies just won't pay for it except when it's used in liquid form during the chemotherapy infusion process. For this reason, for home use, I was given a prescription for Compazine, a less effective but much less expensive antinausea drug that my insurance would cover. Fortunately, it worked well enough.

4. Amniocentesis is a prenatal diagnostic procedure in which a needle is inserted into an expecting mother's abdomen into the uterus and amniotic sac in order to obtain an amniotic fluid sample. The fluid contains cells from the fetus, which can be used to test for genetic and other defects. Amniocentesis is usually done between 15 and 18 weeks of pregnancy.

5. As discussed in chapter 1, neutropenia is a significant decrease in one's neutrophils, the main components of white blood cells, which increases one's risk of infection. It is a common result of blood cancers and chemotherapy.

Chapter 6: "How Can You Know I'm in Remission?"

1. While Neupogen was truly a wonder drug for me and was effective at all stages of the treatment cycle, there is a hypothetical concern that too much Neupogen could cause hematopoietic stem cell exhaustion. This occurs when a person's stem cells proliferate too rapidly, exhausting the regenerative cell pool and making future proliferation slower and more difficult.

2. The process occurs as follows: The original DNA is first heated so that the strands of the double helix separate. Then the reaction is cooled, and primers, which are very short and specific, bind to the complementary strands of the recently separated molecules, and the polymerase takes over, making the rest of the target section of the chain. This procedure—splitting the DNA molecules by heating them and binding the primer with the native and synthesized DNA—is repeated thirty or more times, at which point up to a billion copies of a single section of DNA can be reproduced.

3. The bone marrow transplant that I was to receive was not a full bone marrow transplant; that is, I was not going to have my bone marrow fluid sucked out of my body or killed with chemo and radiation and then have somebody else's healthy bone marrow fluid injected back into me. This is called an allogenic bone marrow transplant. Nor was I to have an allogenic stem cell rescue, an injection of stem cells from a donor matched as closely as possible to my cell types. If all goes well with this type of transplant, the donor's stem or marrow cells will graft into the patient's bones and produce marrow, which will eventually produce the red and white blood

cells and platelets we all need to live. But these marrow and stem cells are also foreign proteins. If a patient's body rejects them (called graft or transplant rejection), nasty drugs that cripple the immune system and make infection likely must be used to train the body to accept them. There is also a high chance of developing graft-versus-host disease, which is the opposite of transplant rejection. In this case, the immune cells in the transplanted stem or marrow cells produce antibodies that attack the patient's own tissue and organs. When this happens, immunosuppressive antirejection drugs, such as cyclosporine, must be administered, which greatly increases a patient's chances of infection and reduces the patient's immune system's capacity to fight cancer naturally. I had the choice between an allo transplant and an "auto transplant" in which my own stem cells would be removed, cleansed, and injected back into my body. The advantage of the allo transplant was that I knew there would not be any cancer cells mixed with the stem or marrow cells from another person—presuming that person didn't have a latent cancer. So the allo transplant would give me a lower probability of losing remission, but there was a greater threat that I wouldn't survive the procedure. That was a cost-benefit trade-off I wasn't willing to make, for the numbers showed that there was about a 30 percent risk of transplant rejection with the allo method. I opted for what I considered to be the least risky transplant: the one in which I would get my own stem cells back after they'd been cleaned of (hopefully all) cancer cells, called an autologous stem cell rescue, or auto transplant. First, my cancer cells would be purged while they were still in my body by the six rounds of chemotherapy plus Rituxan I was to receive, plus an additional chemo known as a mobilization chemo, in which I would be injected with 5,000 milligrams of Cytoxan (compared with the few hundred milligrams I got in each of my CHOPs). The mobilization chemo would drive my immunities to zero, have negative effects on my lungs and heart, and be all-around nasty, but it would reduce the number of cancer cells in my body to a fairly low level. Then I'd be given double-dose injections of Neupogen for a week in order to stimulate what few stem cells were left to multiply like mad—but still, it wouldn't be enough to compensate for all the stem cells I'd lost. In a process known as apheresis, I'd have quite a bit of blood extracted and saved for the stem cell rescue. It would be put through a centrifuge multiple times to separate the midweight cells, which is where most of the stem cells are located, from the other cells. Once they were purged by the centrifuge, the midweight cells would be injected back into my body, and we'd all hope that the stem cells would engraft and that no cancer cells would be injected back into me along with them.

4. A rad, also called a centigray (cGy), is the unit used to describe the dose of radiation being given to a cancer patient. A typical human being's exposure to radiation, both natural and artificial, is about 0.37 rads per year. The amount of radiation in most X-rays is well under 1 rad.

5. Mucositis is an inflammation and ulceration of the mucous membrane (the mucosa) lining the gastrointestinal tract. It is caused when chemotherapy agents or radiation break down the mucosa. Patients may feel pain anywhere along the digestive tract, from the mouth to the anus. Fortunately, the mucosa regenerates rapidly and can grow back in seven to fourteen days in the absence of radiation. Corticosteroid treatment is also effective.

6. My idea for using PCR to test my stem cells that were to be used in the autologous stem cell rescue was this: A primer could be constructed from my tumor sample that was stored in Ron Levy's lab (because I asked for it to be sent there when my biopsy was done). Then, by applying PCR to the stem cell fluid that would later be reinjected into me, we'd be able to find out if there were *any* cancer cells, even one, in the fluid. If we found them, we'd face quite a dilemma about whether to postpone

the rescue, keep purging the stem cells until they were determined to be clean enough, or do an allo transplant instead. However, there was very little information about how the PCR would work and no data against which we could compare my results, violating the frequentist orientation of most of the doctors—and worrying me as well, since I crave frequency data too! But I was nervous about getting my cancer back from my stem cell fluid and was willing to try almost anything that process knowledge suggested was reasonable to reduce the odds of that happening.

7. I had also learned that Sandra's husband, Richard Miller, and the other creators of the machine were sued by Baxter, the drug company, for patent infringement on some horribly specious grounds, like they used computers in designing a cancer machine, and unbelievably, the courts actually backed up that nonsense. Sandra confirmed, and I explained to her that my friends in Europe had told me—and indeed they had, since my Belgian colleague Jean-Pascal van Ypersele has a brother-in-law who worked in a Belgian cancer unit—that Baxter had sold its blood-cleansing machine to a new company, which was marketing an updated version under the name Isolex 300i. I wanted the Isolex 300i used on my stem cells because I was very worried that when my stem cells were removed from my blood for the rescue, a few rogue cancer B cells could still be hanging around with them. What if they were reinjected with the stem cells and I got back the cancer I originally had? That's why the purging of stem cells was so critical, and why all our European colleagues were urging me to press Stanford to start using the Isolex 300i, the machine with the most advanced purging technology. The machine works like a monoclonal antibody works, employing the lock-and-key phenomenon exhibited by a receptor site and a protein. However, unlike the monoclonal antibody (discussed earlier), which causes the patient's immune system to attack its own B cells by making them look like foreign invaders, in the case of the Isolex, a protein binds to the CD-34 receptor site of each stem cell. The protein contains iron, and when it binds to the CD-34 receptor site of the stem cell, the entire stem cell can be attracted to a magnet. The Isolex 300i contains a strong electromagnet, which sucks all the stem cells to one wall of the machine. It then washes the stem cells, releases them, and then reattracts and washes them again. As a result, the Isolex reduces impurities to about one part in 100,000 or 1,000,000, according to our downloads, thereby dramatically lowering the probability that the patient will get his or her cancer back, although it is still not guaranteed to be zero. However, a small number of cancer cells might be below some threshold of risk and might thus be contained by one's own immune system.

Chapter 7: What's So Special About Fifty-Five?

1. As discussed in chapter 5, a multiple gated acquisition, or MUGA, test measures the heart's ejection fraction—the amount of blood the heart pumps out with each contraction.

Chapter 8: Graduation to the Bone Marrow Unit

1. A pulmonary embolism is a blockage of an artery in the lungs, usually by a blood clot, fat, air, or clumped tumor cells.

2. A medical paraprofessional (para, for short) is any medical worker below the level of M.D., including nurses, nurse practitioners, physicians' assistants, nursing aides, and so on.

3. The Isolex 300i would clearly reduce the chances that I would have rogue cancer cells reinjected in the auto transplant or come down with full-blown mantle cell

lymphoma in another year or two, but PCR would tell us if *any* cancer cells were present. I kept asking to have some of my stem cell fluid tested with PCR so we could see whether any cancer cells were left in it, but not even the patient from hell was persistent or persuasive enough to achieve that goal. Anyhow, suppose they did find cancer in my stem cell fluid; what would we have done? More chemos and Rituxan? An allo transplant, assuming we could find a suitable donor in my family or elsewhere? Allo transplants carry a much higher risk of rejection and even death, so I didn't want that, at least not yet. It was another Catch-22, but still, I sure wanted to know if my stem cell fluid had any cancer hiding in it, even if it was only a few cells.

Chapter 9: Zap It to Me: Staring into a Hiroshima-Dose of Radiation

1. Sources: http://www.physics.isu.edu/radinf/risk.htm; and Wilson, R., 1979: "Analyzing the Risks of Daily Life," *Technology Review* 81.
2. A millirem is .001 rem. A rem, or roentgen equivalent man, relates a dose of radiation to its biological effects, whereas a rad (discussed earlier) simply measures the amount of radiation energy transferred to a human being or another mass. To convert from rads to rems or millirems, rads must be multiplied by a quality factor. However, for gamma rays and beta particles, the math is simple: One rad equals one rem. (Source: http://www.stevequayle.com/ARAN/rad.conversion.html.)

Chapter 10: Hospital Arrest

1. Bjorn Lomborg is best known (or most notorious, in scientific circles) for his book *The Skeptical Environmentalist*, in which he contends that the claim made by many natural scientists that a large-scale degradation of the environment is taking place is false, or at least exaggerated. My colleagues and I prepared a rebuttal to various chapters of that book, and it was published in the January 2002 issue of *Scientific American*. I was working on a follow-up.
2. Delaying treatment would be cost-effective because the more time that passes, the cheaper and more effective treatments can become. In addition, we must consider the return on investment. Let's say better diagnostic tests (like a $5,000 PCR test) were performed on a patient. They are worth it in pure monetary terms if they delay a $300,000 bone marrow transplant by only a few years. If we assume a (quite modest) 5 percent per year return on investment, 5 percent of $300,000 is $15,000, so it is very cost-effective to spend $5,000 or $10,000 now to push a bone marrow transplant even one year into the future. For a many-year postponement, it is spectacularly cost-effective to do the PCR diagnostic tests.

Chapter 12: How Much Risk Is Too Much?

1. Atrial fibrillation occurs when the atria—the heart's two smaller upper chambers—quiver rather than beating normally. As a result, blood doesn't get completely pumped out of the atria. This isn't risky in itself; it just makes the heart work harder. The risk is that if the atrial fibrillation is prolonged over a day or more, clots can form in the heart, and when regular sinus rhythm returns, the clots can get blown out and can cause strokes—some potentially life threatening.
2. In the United States in 2003, it was reported that 33,471 occupants of vehicles and 3,661 motorcyclists died in car accidents, of a population of about 290,810,000, which makes for a death rate of about 0.01 percent. In 2003, 4,749 pedestrians were killed in car accidents for a death *rate* of next to nothing—but with a large population

size, even a very small rate means many individuals die. Source: Statistics from the U.S. Department of Transportation's National Highway Traffic Safety Administration, "Motor Vehicle Traffic Crash Fatality Counts and Injury Estimates for 2003" (http://www-nrd.nhtsa.dot.gov/pdf/nrd-30/NCSA/PPT/2003AARelease.pdf).

Chapter 13: Can't I Stay Another Day?

1. Staph (pronounced "staff") is short for *Staphylococcus aureus*. A staph infection occurs when this bacteria enters the body, typically through a cut or other opening in the skin. It is characterized by redness and irritation around a puncture site, swollen lymph nodes, boils or pimples around hair follicles, and persistent cases of strep throat and earaches. A diagnosis is determined by taking a swab of the infected site, culturing it, and testing it. Healthy people typically do not become dangerously ill from staph infections, and they are relieved of them with a simple course of antibiotics, but a staph infection can be devastating to those with weakened immune systems—like cancer patients in treatment. It can spread to the bloodstream, the bones, and the lungs and can cause the joints to swell and permanently stiffen. If it makes it to the lungs, it can cause pneumonia, and if it spreads to the heart, it can cause permanent damage. Sources: Page Wise (http://ilil.essortment.com/whatisastaph_rwaf.htm) and Go Ask Alice! (http://www.goaskalice.columbia.edu/2109.html).

Chapter 15: A Delicate Balance

1. Edema is a swelling, usually of the legs, that results from an accumulation of excess fluid. There are many causes, including prolonged sitting or standing; weakened valves in the veins of the legs, which makes it more difficult for blood to be pumped efficiently back to the heart; chronic lung diseases, such as emphysema and bronchitis, which increase the blood pressure in the blood vessels connecting the heart and lungs, causing higher blood pressure in the right side of the heart; congestive heart failure; and low protein levels in the blood (usually a sign of malnutrition or kidney or liver disease), which causes less salt and water to be retained in the blood vessels and pushes it into the tissues. Sandra was a little concerned that my edema might have had something to do with a weak heart, but after an echocardiogram—another case of proper individualization—it was clear that my heart was not the problem. Rather, it turned out that my blood protein levels were low, which caused fluid to leak through my veins and arteries and into my tissues, triggering the edema. Loss of protein is a common "morbidity" of radiation treatment and bone marrow transplants. Little did I know how significant edema was to become in my life and treatment several years later.

Chapter 16: Size Matters

1. In radioimmunotherapy, a radioactive material is attached to monoclonal antibodies that are designed to target the patient's specific cancer cells. The monoclonal antibodies attach themselves to surface proteins on the cancer cells and deliver the radioactive material directly to the target cells with less damage to healthy tissues.

A GUIDE TO WEB REFERENCES

I found the following Web sites helpful in my own quest for information on my disease. We have also created a Web site for our readers (http://patientfromhell.org), which will include the references below and others as we become aware of them. We will also add news stories relevant to our topics, as well as photos and other items about me.

American Association for Cancer Research
(http://www.aacr.org)
While this site is more geared toward medical professionals, its list of publications may prove helpful to patients.

American Cancer Society
(http://www.cancer.org)
Perhaps the best-known cancer resource on the Web, the American Cancer Society's site is host to valuable information for patients, friends, family, survivors, *and* medical professionals. Their "Interactive Help" section is useful (although it must be remembered that not even the American Cancer Society has all information about the latest clinical trials results).

Cancer Compass
(http://www.cancercompass.com)
This Web site serves as an online community center for cancer patients, supported by the Cancer Treatment Centers of America and the Cancer Treatment Research Foundation (both of which have their own helpful Web sites).

Cancer Guide
(http://www.cancerguide.org)
A cancer survivor provides a wealth of information on cancer statistics, treatments, finance, and so on. Particularly useful are the sections "Researching Your Options" and "Clinical Trials and Experimental Treatments." In the latter, the section "Getting New Treatments Outside a Clinical Trial" is well worth reading.

Cancer Information Service
(http://cis.nci.nih.gov/index.html)
The National Cancer Institute (part of the National Institutes of Health) created this site to provide information on cancer news and resources.

Cancer Survivors Network (American Cancer Society)
(http://www.acscsn.org)
The American Cancer Society maintains this Web site for cancer survivors. It contains survivors' personal accounts of their battles with cancer, chat rooms, information on support groups for survivors, and other useful resources.

iHealthRecord
(http://www.ihealthrecord.org/)
As mentioned in chapter 12, I believe there is a need for more integrated medical care and centralized patient records. If you are concerned that your medical records are not centralized, you may be interested in iHealthRecord. On their Web site, you may enter information about your insurance, emergency contacts, medical conditions, and medications, all free of charge. Your information is always accessible online and can be accessed only with your user name and password. It may be useful to your doctors or in case of emergency, as you could authorize them to log on to your or a loved one's account.

Lymphoma Research Foundation
(http://www.lymphoma.org/)
The Lymphoma Research Foundation is the largest U.S. voluntary health organization focused on lymphoma. It funds a significant amount of lymphoma research and provides valuable information for patients and medical professionals. Of particular interest to patients, their families, and their advocates will be the section of the Web site on Patient Support, which includes information about treatments, support groups, and financial aid.

OncoLink (University of Pennsylvania)
(http://www.oncolink.upenn.edu)
This site gives information on everything from types of cancer to clinical trials to coping with cancer. Check out the OncoLink library for a diversity of reading on cancer.

Patient Advocacy Resources (University of Connecticut Health Center)
(http://library.uchc.edu/departm/hnet/advocacy.html)
The University of Connecticut Health Center library provides a helpful list of patient advocacy books and Web sites.

Patient Advocate Foundation
(http://www.patientadvocate.org)
If you need a case manager or an attorney to act as a liaison between you and your insurance agency, employer, or creditors, see the services offered by the Patient Advocate Foundation detailed on this Web site.

Patient Advocate Liaison Services
(http://www.paliaison.com)
This is the Web site for a professional patient advocate based in Tucson, Arizona. It gives a good overview of what to expect from a patient advocate. It is my hope that such advocates and Web sites will proliferate in the future.

*patient*INFORM.org
(http://www.patientinform.org/)
This site represents a collaboration of voluntary health organizations, scholarly and medical publishers, medical societies, and information professionals. Its goal is to provide patients and caregivers with up-to-date information on and interpretation

of the latest scientific research about their diseases. The three diseases on which the Web site will initially focus are cancer, heart disease, and diabetes. After interpreting new data, the site will give viewers the option to access the full research articles on which the information is based for free.

People Living with Cancer (American Society of Clinical Oncologists)
(http://www.plwc.org)
This Web site provides in-depth resources on cancer types, coping with cancer, and understanding cancer. The "Understanding Cancer" category contains a very useful section, "Communicating With Your Doctor," which gives guidelines for choosing an oncologist and formulating questions to ask him or her, among other things.

The Wellness Community
(http://www.wellness-community.org/default.asp)
Visit this Web site to learn about the Wellness Community, a nonprofit group with twenty-two locations in the United States and two elsewhere providing emotional support and education to cancer patients and their families. Their facilities serve as meeting places and activity centers for cancer patients.

Of course, this is not an exhaustive list of cancer resources available on the Web; there are thousands of pages containing useful information. Once you have received a diagnosis, look up your specific disease on the Web for more information.

ACKNOWLEDGMENTS

This book would not have been possible without the generous support of many, many individuals. I am infinitely grateful to all the doctors and medical staff at Stanford University Medical Center, including Dr. Sandra Horning and her staff, Dr. Michael Jacobs, Dr. Harry Oberhelman, Dr. Ron Levy, Dr. Jeff Petersen, Dr. Karl Blume, Dr. Sean Bohen, Dr. Luis Alvarez, Dr. Natalia Colocci, Dr. Alexandra Simic, Dr. Wenru Song, the radiology team, Dr. James Zehnder and his team, and the wonderful nurses. Without their care, support, and willingness to consider and implement individualized treatments, I might not be here today to write this book. I must also thank Dr. Alessandro Gianni of the Milan Cancer Center for his valuable input regarding treatment after "remission" and Dr. Harvey Fineberg, head of the Institute of Medicine, for critical discussions on applications of decision analysis to medical practices. Thank you to the many people who took the time to read this book and help it progress from rough draft to final product, including my wife Dr. Terry Root, Dr. Donald Kennedy, Dr. Michael Jacobs, Dr. Gary Schoolnik, Dr. Paul Stern, Dr. Warner North, Dr. Alan Garber, and Dr. Richard Miller. I extend my boundless gratitude to my coauthor, Janica Lane, and my editor at the Perseus Books Group, Merloyd Lawrence, who have gone through so many iterations on this book that they can nearly recite it from memory. Finally, many thanks to friends and family, too numerous to name, for their continuing love and support—it really makes a difference.

Abortion, 80
Accidents, 142
Acid reflux, 81
Adriamycin, 74–75
Advocates, 58–60, 77, 79–80, 118, 174, 259, 261, 263, 264
  retired doctors as, 59–60, 259–260
Aflatoxin, 141
Airplanes, 205
Air pollution, 142
Albuterol, 208
Aldo Leopold Leadership program, 232
Allergies, 206, 207, 208, 209, 211, 231. *See also* Chemotherapy, allergic reactions to
Alvarez, Luis, 234–235, 237, 239, 242, 244, 246, 247
American Meteorological Society, 144
Amgen, 7
Amniocentesis, 80
Anesthesia, 48–49, 56, 129, 194
Annals of Oncology, 61
Antibiotics, 3, 154, 159, 164, 184, 194
Anticlotting agents, 182
Anticoagulants, 16, 17, 126, 179, 180
Antifungals, 154, 164–167, 184, 271
Antihistamines, 207
Antinausea drugs, 9, 74, 81, 111
Antivirals, 154, 164, 184
Anxiety, 119, 123, 135, 153, 270

Apheresis, 125, 134–138
Appetite, 81, 82
Armstrong, Lance, 67, 72
Arrhythmias, 51, 208
Asking questions, 8–9, 49, 96–97, 98–103, 120, 257, 259
Aspen, Colorado, 50
Aspirin, 178, 179, 182
Ativan, 152–153
Atrial fibrillations, 178–179, 180
Australia, 34, 35–40
  Greenhouse Office and National University, 36
  Parliamentary Committee on Treaties, 37
Average patient, 116, 140, 146, 176, 257. *See also under* Data issues

Bacteria, 2, 4, 69, 133, 154, 200–201
Bayes, Thomas, 24
Bayesian updating, 9, 11, 24–25, 28, 63, 96, 104, 163, 173, 240, 253, 254, 260
B cell receptors (CD–20), 69–70, 106, 136–137, 226, 241, 246, 249, 251, 253. *See also* Lymphoma, B-cell type
Benadryl, 9–10, 67, 71, 74, 77, 153, 242, 243
Benzopyrene, 141

Biodiversity, 19, 29
Biopsies, 8
    of bone marrow, 8, 55–57, 109–110,
        111, 112, 120, 201–202, 205, 225,
        252, 270
    of colon, 236
    of kidneys, 235, 237
    of lymph nodes, 42, 43–44, 45, 48,
        49, 268
Birds, 39, 155
Blessing-Moore, Dr. Joann, 207, 208
Blood (journal), 222, 256
Blood-brain barrier, 89, 114
Blood clots, 126, 178, 179, 182
Blood platelets, 149, 171, 178, 179
Blood pressure, 8
Blood tests, 2, 3–4, 7, 10, 12, 34, 40, 53,
        92, 132, 192, 210, 212, 263
    blood protein tests, 234, 235, 240,
        241–242, 248
    for lung function, 117–118
    See also White blood cell counts
Blood transfusions, 100, 125, 151, 171
Blume, Dr. Karl, 185–189, 191, 192,
        193, 194, 231
Bohen, Sean, 247
Bone marrow transplant, 58, 88, 89, 93,
        95, 102, 108, 109–110, 112, 113,
        120–121, 164, 171, 185, 206, 212,
        222, 238, 269–270
    allo transplant, 217, 238
    and recovery, 186–187
    See also Cancer, in bone marrow
Brain tumors, 100
Broncospasms, 208, 211, 212
Bush, George W., 35, 221

Calcium, 244, 245, 246
California State University at Chico,
        244–246
Cancer, 8, 264
    activities during treatment for, 145
    alternative/complementary
        treatments, 61–62

    in bone marrow, 61, 77, 79, 185. *See
        also* Biopsies, of bone marrow;
        Bone marrow transplant
    breast cancer, 8, 267
    and DNA abnormalities, 92
    lung cancer, 267
    and median mortality, 64–65
    and proteins coating kidneys, 235
    risks, 141
    stage IV, 61
    and support, 84, 167, 189
    T-cell type, 69
    See also Lymphoma
Carbon dioxide, 26
Caregivers, 84, 126, 189, 267–275
    support for, 271, 272
Carson, Johnny, 175
Cataracts, 93, 118
Center for Evidence-Based Medicine, 104
Chemotherapy, 1–3, 7, 11–12, 53, 55,
        67–84, 85, 91, 102, 111, 222, 253
    allergic reactions to, 9–10, 81
    before bone marrow transplant, 121,
        125, 133, 139, 151
    CHOP protocol, 74, 77, 88, 224,
        254–255, 270
    drip rates, 68, 71, 72
    first chemo session, 4
    and heart ejection fraction, 65
    protocols concerning, 10, 11, 12
    reaction to Rituxan, 72
    side effects, 81–82, 83, 88, 111–112,
        133
    white blood cell cycle between, 3
Chervin, Bob, 144–145
Childhood leukemia, 76
Chlorofluorocarbons, 202
Cholesterol levels, 8
Chronic lymphocytic leukemia, 52
Chronic myeloid leukemia, 250
Civil defense, 150–151
Climate change, 18, 35, 40, 106, 221,
        227–228, 264
    and plants and animals, 14, 18, 28–30

preventive approach to, 19
See also Global warming
Climate science, 15, 25, 27, 36, 144,
209–210. *See also* Environmental
science
Clinical trials, 22–23, 61, 62–63, 90. *See
also* Data issues, clinical trials data
Clotting agents, 149, 171
Coal, 26, 35–36
Colocci, Natalia, 251
Colonoscopy, 235, 236
Compazine, 81, 88, 111
Complex systems, 210
Computer models, 27
Conarton, Sharon, 83
Consensus, 27, 29, 30
Costs, 7–8, 11–12, 34, 38, 60, 127, 132
of antifungals, 166–167, 168
cost-benefit analysis, 12, 13, 19, 77,
101, 105–106, 143, 168, 169, 181,
182, 198, 225–226, 261
of maintenance therapy with
Rituxan, 105, 106
private/social, 12, 169, 170, 264
Coumadin, 179, 180, 181, 182
Crocodile Dundee (film), 36
CT scan, 60, 65, 92, 94, 97, 98–99, 107,
109, 120, 197, 217, 236
Cyclosporine, 239
Cyclotrons, 141
Cytoxan (cyclophosphamide), 74, 77,
111, 121, 133, 151

Daily, Gretchen, 272
Data issues, 21, 22, 250
and average patient, 104, 105, 137,
259
clinical trials data, 62–63, 90, 103,
104, 115, 259. *See also* Clinical
trials
data about maintenance therapy with
Rituxan, 241
data about process, 24, 103–105, 115,
227, 241, 256, 264

frequency data, 22, 23, 24, 25, 54,
70–71, 77, 103–105, 224, 263
historical data, 27, 54, 103
skewed distribution of, 64–65
Decision analysis, 13, 57, 60, 63, 79, 90,
91, 94, 95, 98, 101, 104, 105, 106,
108, 114, 115, 116, 117, 121, 143,
149, 182–183, 198, 257–258,
260–261
Decision flow chart, 98, 99
Decision-making, 28, 60, 77
Deforestation, 26
Demerol, 166
Department of Health and Human
Services, 169
Dermatitis, 206, 207
Developing countries, 15–16, 35
Diuretics, 243–244
DNA, 92
Dreifus, Claudia, 254

Economists, 12, 19, 169
Edema, 206, 207, 211, 231, 233, 234,
235, 239–240, 243
Ehrlich, Paul and Anne, 36, 41, 81, 128,
153, 156, 157, 174, 271
Electrolytes, 243–244
E-mail, 93, 128, 149, 153, 161, 163,
174, 191–192, 198, 250, 257,
271
Emotions, 176–177, 185, 248
Energy Modeling Forum (Aspen), 50,
51, 52
Energy taxes, 20
Environmental science, 13, 175. *See also*
Climate science
Eosinophils, 209, 210
Errors, type I and II, 19–21, 38,
226–227, 227–228. *See also*
Precautionary principle
Etoposide, 152
European health care system, 227
Evidence-based medicine, 104, 105
Exercise, 190, 191

Exhaustion, 81, 111–112
Exponential growth, 254–256

Falsification doctrine, 21, 23
FDA. *See* Food and Drug Administration
Fentanyl, 188, 192, 202–203
Fineberg, Harvey, 63
Fleuriau-Halcomb, Françoise, 5
Flu, 208, 212, 233–234
Food and Drug Administration (FDA), 107, 115
Fossil fuels, 15, 20, 26. *See also* Coal
France, 227
Frequentists. *See* Theorists and frequentists

GDP. *See* Gross domestic product
Genentech biotechnology company, 70, 219
Genetic defects, 80
Geneva, Switzerland, 14, 18, 28
Gianni, Dr. Alessandro, 223–228, 254, 256, 263
Global economy, 19
Global positioning system (GPS), 39
Global warming, 14–16, 19, 20, 29, 30, 35, 36, 37, 40, 47, 208
  role of clouds in, 23
  See also Climate change
Gould, Stephen Jay, 64–65
Goulder, Larry, 275
GPS. *See* Global positioning system
Graft-versus-host disease, 238
Greenhouse effect, 15, 35. *See also* Climate change; Global warming
Gross domestic product (GDP), 19, 169
Grumman Aviation, 154, 156
Gums, 161

Hadley, Liz, 272
Hair loss, 84, 206
Health care legislation, 60, 169, 170, 260
Health care spending, 169

Health insurance. *See* Medical insurance
Heart ejection fraction, 65, 117–118
Heart rhythms, 243, 244. *See also* Arrhythmias
HEPA. *See* High-efficiency particulate air filter discs
Heparin, 126, 130
Heritage sites, 19
Hickman catheters, 124–133, 146, 149, 154, 184
  Hickman hygiene, 126, 130
  removing, 161, 193–194
  technicians for, 128
High-efficiency particulate air (HEPA) filter discs, 123, 152, 156–158, 195–196, 197, 198, 200
HMOs, 34, 60, 169, 258, 261, 264. *See also* Medical insurance
Horning, Dr. Sandra, 1, 5, 10–11, 51, 52–53, 56–57, 58, 60–61, 65, 78, 81, 89, 90, 91, 94–95, 97–103, 107–108, 109, 113–114, 139, 197–198, 200, 223, 229–230, 236–237, 240–241
  advocating maintenance therapy, 252–253
  and change in protocol, 108, 114–115, 260
  change in relationship with, 108, 124, 198, 253
  Fellow assisting, 53–55, 94, 110, 112–113, 120, 207, 247, 251, 269
  and PCR, 203–204, 210–211, 214–215, 216, 217, 220, 237, 249, 253, 254
Hospitals, 34, 96, 119, 121, 258, 261, 264
  clean rooms, 151, 152, 154–156, 187
  and clinical trials data, 63
  and decision sciences, 183
  medication errors in, 159–160
  teaching hospitals, 43, 182

Howard, John, 35, 36
Humor, 135
Hydroxydaunorubicin
(doxorubicin/Adriamycin),
74–75
Hyperactivity, 81

IDEC Pharmaceuticals, 69, 70
Immune system, 2, 69–70, 73, 78, 100,
102, 123, 133, 154, 164, 186, 187,
206, 207, 215, 216, 229
Individualization of diagnosis/treatment,
170, 256, 257, 259, 260, 261,
262–263, 264
partial individualization, 262
Indonesia, 35
Industrialization, 15, 26
Infections, 2, 4, 6, 102, 131, 164, 165,
187, 197, 208, 229, 271
staph infection, 193–194
Injections, 85–86, 126, 132, 166
Institute of Medicine, 63, 160
Integrated medical care, 181
Interest groups, 20
Intergovernmental Panel on Climate
Change (IPCC), 14, 17, 20, 21, 26,
27, 37
Assessment Report, 18
plenary meeting in Geneva, 28–32
Summary for Policy Makers, 30–32
Working Groups I and II, 18
Internet, 52, 61–62, 63, 96, 120, 262,
270
Interventional radiology, 128
Intestinal problems, 4, 184, 191, 200
IPCC. See Intergovernmental Panel on
Climate Change
Island states, 19
Isolex 300i blood-cleansing machine,
107, 114–115, 122, 223, 263
IVs, 9, 48, 71, 74, 135–138

Jacobs, Dr. Michael, 17, 33–34, 40,
45–46, 47, 51–52, 178, 182, 234

Journal of the American Medical
Association, 62

Kidneys, 216, 234, 235, 238–239, 247,
248
Knowing vs. not knowing, 78–80, 83–84
Kyoto Protocol, 35, 36, 37, 221
Kytril, 74

Lasix, 243, 244
Learning curves, 27
Lederman, Leon, 141
Left brain, 2, 11–12, 47, 112, 116, 147,
156, 159, 176–177, 182
Leukemia, 52, 76, 93, 101, 102, 118,
143, 250
Levy, Ron, 48, 49, 69, 93, 97, 103, 198,
226, 229
Lidocaine, 56, 208, 270
Liem, Dr. L. Bing, 180–181, 182
Life expectancy, 270. See also Mortality
rates
Lindzen, Richard, 37, 38, 47
Liver, 81, 88, 91, 119, 136, 139, 141
Lollies, 161, 162, 177, 184, 191, 202
Lomborg, Bjorn, 162
Lovejoy, Tom, 41, 44, 76
Lubchenco, Jane, 233
Lungs, 6, 102, 116, 117–118, 139, 140,
147, 148, 165, 232
allergic reactions in, 208–209, 210,
211
Lymphoma, 1
B-cell type, 7, 45, 54, 69, 240, 256.
See also B cell receptors
first indications of, 16–17, 33, 40, 41,
267
indolent/aggressive, 54, 88
life expectancy for, 270
mantle cell lymphoma, 13, 54, 57,
61, 69, 88, 138, 222, 223, 253,
269, 270
recovery, 186–189, 192
support groups for, 52

Lymphoma (*continued*)
treatment/protocols for, 20, 51, 57,
86, 91, 94, 95, 96, 108, 114, 222,
223–224, 270. *See also*
Chemotherapy, CHOP protocol;
Maintenance therapy

Madagascar periwinkle, 75
Maintenance therapy, 88–91, 92–93,
102, 103, 105, 197–198, 201, 215,
217, 218, 219, 220, 225–226, 228,
229, 231, 236–237, 239, 240–241,
246–247, 254, 255–256, 263
Rituxan doses stretched out over a
year, 252–253
Maldives, 19
Mallee fowls, 39–40
Mearns, Linda, 144
Media, 21
"Median Isn't the Message, The"
(Gould), 64–65
Medical errors, 160
Medical insurance, 34, 38, 66
insurance companies, 60, 127,
169–170, 258, 264
and patient advocacy, 260
See also HMOs
Medical schools, 105, 258
Medical testing, 7–9, 13, 127
waiting for results of, 118, 119–120,
135
See also Blood tests; Polymerase chain
reaction; Urine tests
Medicine by the book/numbers, 4,
12–13, 116, 173
Melanoma, 216
Membranous glomerulonephritis (MG),
238, 239, 240, 241, 242
Methane, 26
MG. *See* Membranous
glomerulonephritis
Microbiology, 91, 106
Milan, Italy, 221, 223
Miller, Richard, 69, 107

Minimal residual disease (MRD), 106,
222, 240, 247, 252
Monoclonal antibody, 69, 70, 106, 136
Mood changes, 82
Morphine, 160–161, 162–164, 173, 184,
188, 271
Mortality rates, 57, 64–65, 141–142,
270
and medical errors in hospitals, 160
Mourning, 177, 185
MRD. *See* Minimal residual disease
Mucositis, 100–101, 149, 161, 162, 163,
184, 191
MUGA. *See* Multiple gated acquisition
scan
Multiple gated acquisition (MUGA)
scan, 65, 117–118
Murdock, Rick, 107
Myeloablative action, 77, 121

Naps, 191, 192, 199
Nausea, 81, 83, 88, 110, 111. *See also*
Antinausea drugs
National Academy of Sciences, 202
National Cancer Institute, 61
National Center for Atmospheric
Research (NCAR), 143–145
National Committee for Quality
Assurance, 160
NCAR. *See* National Center for
Atmospheric Research
Nephrotic syndrome, 234–235, 238
Neupogen, 7, 11–12, 85–86, 91, 117,
134, 136, 168, 171–173, 263
Neutropenia, 4–5, 81
Neutrophil count, 4–5, 11, 103
New York Times, 254
Nonlinear systems, 209–210
Northern Exposure (television show),
164, 274
Novocain, 203, 237
Nuclear war, 150–151
Nurses, 159–160, 162–163, 174, 189,
200–201, 205

Oberhelman, Dr. Harry, 42, 45, 47, 49–50
Oncologists, progressive vs. traditional, 254
Oncovin. *See* Vincristine
OPEC nations, 15
Out-of-body experiences, 58, 87

Patient Number One (Murdock), 107
PCR. *See* Polymerase chain reaction
Peripheral neuropathy, 76, 133, 188, 190, 231, 232
Perle, Richard, 150
Petersen, Dr. Jeff, 234, 237, 239, 246
PET scan, 60, 65–66
Phlebitis, 16, 17
Pitelka, Lou, 52
Placebos, 103
Pneumonia, 4
Policy issues in climate change, 18–19, 26, 35, 221
  wait-and-see policy, 37
Polymerase chain reaction (PCR), 91–92, 107, 113, 122, 138, 197, 201, 218–219, 222, 223, 224–225, 231, 247, 248, 256, 263
  noise level for, 250–251, 252
  tests on blood vs. tissues, 251–252
  use in Europe, 227
  See also Horning, Dr. Sandra, and PCR
Potassium, 244, 245, 246
Precautionary principle, 20, 36–38, 227, 256, 261. *See also* Errors, type I and II
Predator-prey situations, 255–256
Prednisone, 74, 78, 85, 110, 207, 208, 211, 239, 240
  withdrawal from, 82–83, 86–87
Probabilities, 20, 21, 22, 23, 57, 80, 91, 105, 110, 180, 272
  cognitive psychology on estimating, 101
  confidence levels of probability judgments, 27
  and PCR, 213–214

prior and revised-prior probability, 25. *See also* Bayesian updating
  See also Subjective probability analysis
Process knowledge. *See* Data issues, data about process
Pulmonary embolism, 126
Pushnik, Jim, 245

Questions. *See* Asking questions

Radiation illness, 150–151, 152, 162
Radiation treatment, 89, 98, 142, 222, 255
  lead plates for, 139, 140, 143, 147
  radiation risk, 142–143
  and static electricity effect, 147
  whole body radiation, 99–102, 108, 114, 116–118, 121, 140, 263
  X-rays vs. electron beams, 140–141, 148
  See also Side effects, of radiation
Radioimmunotherapy, 217
Rashes, 206–208, 211, 212, 239
Regression model, 172
Remission, 89, 90, 92, 98–99, 109, 143
  vs. cure, 100
  full remission, 109–115, 124, 128
  molecular/clinical remission, 222, 255, 256
  remission rates for Dr. Gianni's protocol, 223–224
Renewable energy, 15, 20
Research protocols, 115, 201, 202, 203
Reverse placebo effect, 78, 79
Riccelli, Angela, 272, 274–275
Risk assessment, 23, 25–28, 38, 105, 141–143, 258
Rituxan, 68–69, 70–74, 77, 78, 111, 136, 165, 228–229, 254–255, 270
  costs, 105, 106
  for MG treatments, 239–243, 247, 248, 263
  See also Maintenance therapy

Rituximab, 70
Root, Terry L., 2, 6–7, 11, 14–15, 16,
    28, 34, 36–37, 39–40, 44, 46, 47,
    49, 53, 55, 56, 59, 71–72, 83–84,
    85–86, 93, 95–96, 107, 167,
    173–174, 185, 213, 222, 238,
    271
    Afterword by, 267–275
Rosencranz, Armin, 198

Saving Private Ryan (film), 58
Schneider, Becca and Adam, 50, 167
Scientific American, 162
Scientific theory, 21–22
Side effects, 28, 48, 50, 57, 80, 206
    of antifungals, 165–166, 168
    of bone marrow transplant, 206,
        212
    of Coumadin, 180, 181
    of Cytoxan, 77
    of Neupogen, 86
    of radiation, 99–102, 108, 116, 140,
        146, 149
    of Rituxan, 229
    of vincristine, 76–77
    See also under Chemotherapy
Smoking, 141, 267
Solomon, Susan, 202
Spiegel, David, 84
Standard of living, 26, 76
Stanford University Medical Center, 1,
    33, 40, 47
    bone marrow unit, 123, 192, 193,
        200, 202
    dermatology unit, 207
    Fellows at, 193, 218, 219, 234. See
        also Horning, Doctor Sandra,
        Fellows assisting
    infusion room in, 242
    nephrology unit, 234
    new protocol for mantle cell
        lymphoma at, 57, 86, 108, 114. See
        also Chemotherapy, CHOP
        protocol

Oncology Day Care Center, 3, 5, 7,
    53, 94, 98, 202, 268
Statistics, 64–65
Stem cells, 86, 88, 107, 108, 115, 122,
    125, 133–134, 135–138. See also
    Bone marrow transplant;
    Polymerase chain reaction
Steroids, 78, 207, 208, 212
Stress hormones, 220
Stroke, 179, 180, 182
Subjective probability analysis, 24, 37,
    104, 261. See also Bayesian
    updating; Probabilities
Superior vena cava, 125, 126, 194
Support, 52, 94, 128, 175, 268, 271,
    275. See also under Cancer;
    Caregivers
Surgery, 42–43, 45, 48, 49
Symposia, 273–274

Taste, altered sense of, 83–84
T cells, 239
Temperature (of individuals), 110, 191,
    192–193, 194, 232, 233
Tests. See Blood tests; Medical testing;
    Polymerase chain reaction; Urine
    tests
Theorists and frequentists, 22–24
Tonight Show, 175
Total parenteral nutrition (TPN), 184
TPN. See Total parenteral nutrition
Transitioning, 186
Triage, 260
Tropical forests, 76
Tuvalu, 19
Tylenol, 233

Ultrasound, 40
Uncertainty, 27, 28, 258
    deep uncertainty, 20, 23, 106, 115, 264
    in science of global warming, 36, 37
United Nations, 18, 29
    Conference on Environment and
        Development (1992), 26

Framework Convention on Climate
    Change, 221
Urine tests, 2354, 235, 240, 241–242,
    247–248

Vaccinations, 38
Value judgments, 80–81
Versed, 48–49, 49–50, 129, 236
Vesicants, 74–75, 111
Vicodin, 134
Vincristine, 75–77, 111, 133
VP–16 (myeloablative drug), 121, 152,
    153

Wall, Diana, 46
Watson, Robert, 31–32
Weakness, 191
Web. *See* Internet

White blood cell counts, 10, 86, 91,
    119, 134, 136, 155, 159, 171,
    175–176, 181, 185, 200, 201, 205,
    209, 210, 211–212
    and pain increase, 172–173
    nadir point, 2, 3, 6
Wine, 81, 83, 119, 128, 136, 141
World Meteorological Organization, 18
Wynbrandt, Gary, 82–83, 176–177, 202,
    248

X-rays, 156

Yoffe, Gideon, 272
Yogurt, 200–201

Zehnder, Dr. James, 249–250, 251
Zithromax, 232

ABOUT THE AUTHORS

Stephen H. Schneider of Stanford University is a climatologist and professor in the Department of Biological Sciences, a Senior Fellow at the Institute for International Studies, and Professor by Courtesy in the Department of Civil and Environmental Engineering. Schneider was elected to the US National Academy of Science in 2002 and received the National Conservation Achievement Award from the National Wildlife Foundation and the Edward T. Law Roe Award of the Society of Conservation Biology in 2003. In 1992, he was awarded a MacArthur Prize Fellowship. He disseminates his message not only to students, but also to the general public, other scientists, and political figures through public lectures, seminars, classroom teaching, environmental assessment committees, media appearances, Congressional testimony, and research collaboration with colleagues. Schneider founded the journal *Climatic Change* in 1975 and serves as its editor. His books include *The Co-evolution of Climate and Life*, *Encyclopedia of Climate and Weather*, *Climate Change Policy: A Survey*, and *Wildlife Responses to Climate Change*.

For more information see http://www.patientfromhell.org.

Janica Lane is a research assistant to Stephen Schneider. She received undergraduate degrees in International Relations and Spanish from Stanford in 2000. Lane began working for Professor Schneider in 2003, focusing on extensive research and writing related to climate change and to cancer.